LIFE'S WORK

A Memoir

DAVID MILCH

RANDOM HOUSE

NEW YORK

Published in the United States by Random House, an imprint and
division of Penguin Random House LLC, New York.

RANDOM HOUSE and the HOUSE colophon are registered
trademarks of Penguin Random House LLC.

LIBRARY OF CONGRESS CATALOGING-IN-PUBLICATION DATA
Names: Milch, David, author.
Title: Life's work: a memoir / David Milch.
Description: First edition. | New York: Random House, 2022.
Identifiers: LCCN 2022004572 (print) | LCCN 2022004573
(ebook) | ISBN 9780525510741 (hardcover) |
ISBN 9780525510758 (ebook)
Subjects: LCSH: Milch, David, 1945- | Television writers—
United States—Biography. | Television producers and directors—
United States—Biography.
Classification: LCC PN1992.4.M555 A3 2022 (print) |
LCC PN1992.4.M555 (ebook) | DDC 791.4302/32092
[B]—dc23/eng/20220503
LC record available at https://lccn.loc.gov/2022004572
LC ebook record available at https://lccn.loc.gov/2022004573

Photographs on pages 25 and 55 are by William Ferris,
William R. Ferris Collection, Southern Folklife Collection,
The Wilson Library, University of North Carolina at Chapel Hill.

Printed in Canada on acid-free paper

randomhousebooks.com

2 4 6 8 9 7 5 3 1

FIRST EDITION

Book design by Simon M. Sullivan

To my beloved brother Bob, who I miss every day.

Tell me a story.

In this century, and moment, of mania,
Tell me a story.

Make it a story of great distances, and starlight.

The name of the story will be Time,
But you must not pronounce its name.

Tell me a story of deep delight.

—Robert Penn Warren

Prologue

I'M ON A BOAT SAILING TO SOME ISLAND where I don't know anybody. A boat someone is operating, and we aren't in touch.

Sometimes if you've been unwell and in the hospital and they aren't yet sure what's wrong with you, waiting to find out what tests have to be done for them to understand what's wrong, you experience that fundamental uncertainty about the state of your relation to the world. Am I about to leave it? You feel so provisional in your connection to what you're experiencing.

I'm losing my faculties. Things seem a continuous taking away. Wake, don't know if it's night or day, or whether to trust the processes of your own body to function. You're not sure where you are, obsessively rehearse what you think might be your obligations, to be certain you're remembering what you need to do or know. You act like you know what someone is talking about when you have no fucking idea. You're just impersonating who you used to be.

My brain has amyloid plaque, they can number how much. The plaques compound. Palliatives slow the spread but nothing arrests it.

I get up at three in the morning, defiantly night. Even the dogs have different personalities. It's a growing solitude. I wonder, and not infrequently, "Is it gone for good?" My mind. And the only answer you get is an answer in that moment. It doesn't hold on. But that's the whole human contract. Seen so, all of this is gone already. Somebody's dealing and you have no choice but to play.

So to take on at this juncture, under these circumstances, the challenge of trying to see things as clearly as possible, identify certain recurring patterns and joys and tragedies, is a blessing. It increasingly seems that life is something that happens to you and art the opportunity to understand what's transpired. You need only to be brave.

I'm intimidated and concerned about limitations my health will impose on writing this book, an ongoing process of discovery. Compounding the intrinsic solitude is the deterioration of a sense of readiness and organization, so there's a necessary continuous reconstitution. Of the process of composition, Robert Penn Warren wrote, "This is the process whereby pain of the past in its pastness may be converted into the future tense of joy." And what he's talking about is this process in which, in its seeming irrecoverability, every kind of pain, brought once again to life, is transformed.

Though I'd be grateful to accomplish some overview or summation, I flinch from that presumption. The patterns and urgencies and imperatives will reveal themselves. The very idea of not knowing as an organizing principle is to be accepted with a proper humility—that it's a privilege not to know and be given a chance to find out. You're always aware there's an irreducible mystery that at best you're going to approach but never going to capture. And reverence for the mystery is itself the organization of the story. My story.

Writing for television rewards the balancing of runners—stories initiated in earlier episodes—with material generated within the episode at hand. Those concerns can be extrapolated into much larger themes about the relation of the past to the present. I imagine there will be some of that here. Certain reoccurrences and repetitions. Also, I'm losing my mind, so that might account for some of it.

At points as you read you might think, "Well, pretty good recall for a guy with Alzheimer's," so I should clarify here that in many cases it's not my current recollection, but a past recollection of mine being shared with me now by my family, who are helping me compose this book. About twenty years ago, my wife began a practice of having my writing process recorded and then having all of the recordings transcribed. We have been going through those materials, pulling out different pieces and moving them around, telling the story together. That is not so different from how I've written most things—in many drafts, through collaboration, over time. My collaborators now being my family, my wife and children, is its own gift in this process. It will also necessarily alter what might have been had I done it alone. I have struggled to notice what's happening around me throughout my life, so in that sense their witness has also provided useful clarification. After John Milton lost his eyesight, he would dictate to his daughters and they would write it down. That's how he wrote *Paradise Lost*. We don't know what happened in that exchange either. Would that it were only my eyes.

We know nothing comes easily in terms of being loyal both to the past and the present. To show the proper weight of the past as it's experienced in the present and how the present goes on, on its own terms—that's the most difficult challenge in the world. Without getting too metaphysical, the weight of the distances and differences that time makes between characters as they're experienced in the present is inevitably the proper theme of storytelling.

There's a poem by T. S. Eliot:

> We shall not cease from exploration
> And the end of all our exploring
> Will be to arrive where we started
> And know the place for the first time.

Contents

LIFE'S
WORK

1.

Peace Bridge

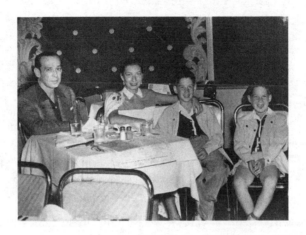

My folks were married when my mom was twenty-two, young for sure. My dad was, relatively speaking for that day and age, senior, at thirty-four.

Mom was a small-town girl, grew up in Batavia, about forty miles outside of Buffalo. Very provincial. Her parents had a furniture store adjoining their house so my grandfather would just walk out one door and in another. The store's still around. There were six children of whom she was the baby. She had four brothers and a sister. That was an identifiable dynamic—she was spoiled and they were all very protective of her. The boys were much less cosmopolitan than the girls. Batavia in those days, ten thousand people, wasn't a city at all. There was that fierce parochialism that you get in a small town. They were defensive—*sure, it's a small town, but I'm big enough to beat your balls off.* They were very close as a family unit.

My dad, and in turn my brother and I, came from a clannish background. It was a knock-around neighborhood my dad grew up in in Buffalo. Tough neighborhood, very much segregated by ethnic groups—Jews were all in one place, Italians in another. His mom, Esther, was the eldest of seven children, though sometimes when I tell this story I say ten children. My dad was an only child. His mom kept having miscarriages because she was diabetic. My dad weighed like sixteen pounds when he was born, too much sugar. Not too long after, Esther's mother croaked—my dad's grandmother. So Esther moved back into her parents' house, and, depending upon how one interprets the data, possibly into her newly widowed father's bed. I think his name was Jacob. The odd man out was her husband, Morris, my grandfather, who had moved into the house with them. Whatever was going on so radically disempowered him that he tried to kill himself by going over Niagara Falls. They have various impediments in place to keep one from accomplishing that feat. He thought he could beat them, but he couldn't. One suspects it wasn't much fun for my dad either.

His grandfather Jake, my great-grandfather, whose bed my dad's mother, Esther, may or may not have been sharing, was not a nice man. Probably his most endearing characteristic was that he was a bootlegger. All the boys in the family—my dad's uncles, my great-uncles—were enlisted one way or another to assist him. During Prohibition, what you never wanted to do was collar a really powerful man. What you wanted to do was collar a miserable Jewish prick, so the cops came to collar my great-grandfather Jake, and he said, "My son did it!" So one of my uncles had to leave town and ended up living on a houseboat in international waters. I think there was a warrant out for him. We'd visit on the docks and he'd stay on his boat. Another uncle started running a joint in Saratoga, the Piping Rock, a casino. When my dad was seventeen or so, he worked there for the summer as a busboy, and he loved it. But because my dad was the next generation, the edict was he had to go to college, so he couldn't be involved in nefarious activities. Nobody was allowed to shoot pool with him. Nobody was allowed to do anything bad with him because he had to go to college. One day one of my uncles comes up to the pool hall, and my dad's shooting pool with a guy. My uncle took the guy, threw him through a window, and broke his neck. He never played pool with my dad again. He never walked again.

What the people of the family said about my dad was, "Elmer can't get involved in what we're involved in." So between that, and whatever the hell had gone on in that house, I think he experienced some sense of otherness, lost what might have been the natural environment for his childhood, or felt that he was being deprived of or cut off from the environment in which he grew up, even as he was growing up there, that he was in a house that was not his own. My dad became a doctor, a surgeon. He published papers. But clearly Saratoga and the racetrack were associated in his mind with a lot of unresolved stuff. And every August he would go back.

My mother used to say he was a small-town boy from a big city. My dad was a good catch. He was a Jewish doctor, older, what's not to like? Besides the flagrant philandering? He was a hard player, drank a lot. He had residual consequences from a terrible car accident. Every three months for thirty, forty years he had to have dilatations, put a rod up his penis, used catheters and sounds to get the urine out.

I could make a number of choices in how I tell the story of

my dad's car accident. He was on an army base where he was a medic and flipped a truck. He was drunk, supposed to ship out the next day, and out to see a woman. The accident got him caught wrong by my mom. I was conceived when he was in the hospital after. I've told the story a lot of different ways. I'm not sure any of it is true.

Now the particulars of my condition make it quite literal that I don't know anymore what parts of the story are true, and what are just parts of different stories I've told. But we're all making choices in how we tell the story and one thing I would suggest is that what literally happened need not be overly determinative.

I was born in 1945. You may know it as a rather significant year in world history. In my experience it's most important as the year I was born. And you wonder why baby boomers fucked everything up.

My mother, Mollie, was content being a mother, but she had done very well in college, got a degree in education, and started to teach. It was a meaningful career for her. My mom lectured, then she became a political figure in Buffalo as head of the city's board of education. They wanted her to run for mayor and my dad said no. I don't know whether she had the temperament to go out and glad-hand the way you have to do. I think she would have, but she had to take care of him. My mom shaped what I was going to do and how I was going to do it, scholastically and all around. She was extremely high performing, always in the pages of our newspaper for her accomplishments. When she was head of the board of education she coined the phrase "It's ten o'clock, do you know where your children are?" The irony being, of course, that she herself never did.

Dad always had a Cadillac, and if there was a rattle or something it would drive him crazy. We lived in fear and dread that the car would make any noise. I've wondered if he had some kind of bipolarity, but I never saw him manic. More unipolar, but not solely depressed. Compulsive. Some people defy diagnosis.

He refused to meet a new person and would come up with the most idiotic explanations of why I couldn't bring a friend over: "No, no, no, no, no, that's bullshit. I don't need that shit. I don't need it. No."

Once a friend of mine fell and split his skull open. I had to bring him home so my dad could stitch him up, and then he wouldn't let the kid leave.

"These are what we call Jewish forks and these are Jewish knives and this is Jewish food."

The kid was baffled.

My dad wanted so much to be open but was so self-enclosed. Alcoholics in particular are like that, everything's got to be exactly the same. Maybe one time out of four in a week my dad would get his oiler on and if he was in a particularly gaseous, effusive mood, he would open the doors to the heathen Gentile.

One year we'd been to Yom Kippur services at Kleinhans Music Hall. The temple population at that time was about two thousand and it would fill the harmonic hall. We had taken the car down early in the day so Dad would have a good parking spot and he could leave quickly. Then we took one cab home to wait, and another back in time for the start of the service. After it was over, we come out of the synagogue and the Caddy's boxed in by an Imperial LeBaron. On Yom Kippur, when all your sins have just been forgiven, Dad reverses hard into the LeBaron—*bang!* Then he pulls up again, reverses—*bang!* Mom is hysterical. But we get out of the space eventually and he's away before everybody else comes out and he can be held responsible. There's always next Yom Kippur to deal with this one.

Rabbi Fink was the boss over at Beth Zion. When God spoke, he spoke through Joe Fink. There was just no question. Everybody in the community respected him. After a bar mitzvah, it was known that the rabbi would place his hands on your shoulders and impart some great wisdom. After mine, I just remember being profoundly disappointed. I can't remember what he said, only the hole remains, but it's still open and still able to generate dissatisfaction. "Thank you very much," I managed. "See you at the reception." It was right about then I understood that adults don't know much either. By thirteen, I was already feeling pretty outside of most things, and you convince yourself that everyone else is inside.

My parents' attitude about Judaism was largely derived from my grandparents. My mom's mother and father were Orthodox, very observant. My older brother Bob's bar mitzvah was their first experience in a Reform temple. We were sitting in the front row of this ornate, Romanesque synagogue. First of all, the men are sitting with the women. Then, the organ starts to play. Just as the choir begins singing on this balcony, my grandmother Anna turns to my mother and says in Yiddish, "When comes the priest?" Two years later my grandparents chose not to attend mine.

I remember Mom, an active Democrat and egalitarian, saying, "Do not bring a goyishe girl home. Don't kill me." We had a lot of Jewish refugees stay with us. My parents used to bore the shit out of me saying everything that happened to anyone who was Jewish was because they were Jewish. "They're screwing them over because they're Jewish." I'm thirteen and I'm saying, "That's nuts." But six million Jews were killed and my parents were alive when that happened. They were hypervigilant. I hadn't had that experience, and so I thought that's crazy. My mother tried to tell me, "You can be friends with a goy, you can be the best friends in the world, but when push comes to shove, a goy will try to kill you." Those admonitions were grotesque, and I choose now to interpret them as a gift in their grotesquerie which was so absolutely refuted by the conduct of the person who uttered them. They were a gift from God to show me: *Don't listen to what people say. Watch only what they do.*

* * *

My dad was always very mysterious about money. The only time I would see money at all was up in Saratoga in August. The first time I was taken to the races my old man says, "I know what you want, because you're a degenerate fucking prick and you got to gamble. You're five years old. You want me to bring you out here. Well, you can't gamble because you're five. You can't bet, but I set it up with Max the waiter and he'll run your bets for you." Within a few years, my dad would have me run his bets for him at the window.

So we come by our tics honestly.

While my parents were in Saratoga, my dad would send us to Camp Paradox, which was nearby in the Adirondacks. It was called that because in the summer the current in the lake flowed one way and the rest of the year it went the other way. I went to that camp for seven or so years, starting when I was six. It wasn't a pleasant place for me. There were behaviors demonstrated by certain adults that undermined my capacity to trust the world—what little capacity I had. Sexual predation and the like. I became closely acquainted with profound feelings of guilt and shame. But on the whole one wouldn't have had it any other way. Because one can't. These are things that happened. I try to feel that way, anyway.

My parents would send a car to pick me up and I would go to the racetrack and be driven back to camp after. Just before I went back, my dad would grab my shirt collar and say, "Don't let me see you sneaking out here."

My relationship with my father was cloaked in secrets and taboos. On Saturday nights we'd go to basketball games at Memorial Auditorium, and there was a guy named Bozo who ran my father's bets. If you ever saw him, you'd know why they called him Bozo—he looked exactly like Bozo the Clown. He was a nice guy. With all the attendant compulsion and drive, I'd run the bets up to Bozo and everything was undercover.

I felt outward as a kid. In certain circumstances, I still think I am. My brother, Bob, stayed at camp and I would go to the track. Bob was more classically inward, which served him. My brother was going to be a doctor, he had been selected for that. I had been selected to be the bum. A version of my dad separated into each of us. There was a sense in which my dad was an elusive presence, in that he was a surgeon and a professor of surgery, and then there was this whole other life that he led. So when I started to exhibit symptoms of degeneracy, it pleased my dad. Although it was also a subject of contumely.

I got sick when I was seven maybe. My appendix burst inside of me. My dad set me up with a television set in the hospital room and he had them wire in the horse-racing channel so I could make bets. "It's just entertainment!" He'd come down between surgeries and sit with me. I spent more time with my father when I was in the hospital than I did when I was outside.

I was always acting out, trying to entertain. One of my mother's brothers had a big nightclub in Miami Beach called La Vie en Rose. We would spend a week in Florida. They'd put me up on the stage and have me sing and I would imitate Jerry Lewis. I wanted to do it because I thought my dad wanted me to do it. It was awful.

When I was eight years old, I stole my first booze. There was always plenty of it in the house. I had compulsions I didn't know what to do with. I had to touch my pillow a certain number of times. I had to move my shoes a certain number of times. I had to tell my parents I love them a certain number of times. I became convinced that my grandfather, whom I had been brought in to kiss when he was dead, used to take one step from his grave every night, and when he finally got to where I was, I would die. So I would keep him busy. I'd move in patterns.

I did my first writing then too, though I didn't know that's what I was doing. I'd take the newspaper and look at the box scores for the baseball games and I'd make up my own radio call for the whole game. Sitting there drunk and alone wearing my dad's hat, reconstructing each of the plays, two different voices calling the game.

Not only was my old man a drinker, but he had a predilection for Demerol. He got hooked when he had been in the hospital after the auto accident. When someone married into the family, he'd rejoice in having another patient for whom to write phony prescriptions.

I was never, during my childhood proper, particularly interested in horses, though I was intrigued by the statistical aspect of racing itself. Our family would eat a very late supper, as my father would go to sleep immediately upon his return from the hospital and not awaken until perhaps ten o'clock. I ate much earlier, but I was required to sit at the table while my father ate. During the course of one of these meals the subject of the opening of the Saratoga racing season arose.

"Saratoga season starts July thirtieth," I said.

"August third," he said.

I had happened to see the date in the paper a few days before and was quite insistent that my date was correct.

"You might know something about baseball, but horse racing is my province. The first day of the meeting is on the third."

He made it clear there was to be no further discussion about it.

So I did not dispute the matter further, but instead went and got the paper and showed him that I was right. There ensued an examination in which I was questioned concerning what horses had won the Triple Crown, who was the only filly to win the Derby, and the like. As I recall I did not know the answer to a single question, nor was I able to offer even a guess. For the next month I forsook the sports pages for the detailed perusal of my father's extensive racing library. It started there, on that night at that dinner table, this need to master it.

My father was partnered with my uncle Chatz (emphasis on the phlegm) whose real name was Harry Levint, and he was a bookmaker and a very effective personality. Chatz was a gangster. He used to punctuate his sentences with, "Y'hear?" I would record his bets too. My uncle Chatz would call and he'd never say the name of the team, just "the favorite" or "the underdog," or he'd run through a whole bet and then say "the opposite." He wasn't really our uncle, but he was Dad's closest non-medical friend. He described himself as a collector of overdue accounts and adjuster of attitudes.

Chatz was very protective toward my dad in terms of what he would permit my dad to get involved in and what was verboten. The mobsters would pick up my dad and take him to operate, remove bullets. That was a big part of my dad's nature, being in the underworld. He felt, I think, constrained by his profession. He was a very well-known doctor, and well respected, but there was an excess of energy, a risk-taking, in what he did. He could have been thrown out of being a physician or arrested at any moment. Being adjacent to the criminal world was a way to satisfy that excess of energy.

In alcoholic families, there's someone called the designated patient, which is one person who is identified as suffering from the disease so that everyone can be talking about him. "He was out again last night, I don't know what the fuck—I shouldn't say I was going through his pants, but I happened to see there's a summons in his pocket. So, it's the same bullshit." What that allows is they don't have to talk about the real problem, which is Dad or whatever else it is. The designated patient's role in the family is to be the sufferer who is out in the open, and to distract the outside world from paying attention to the real sufferer in the family. My job in our family was to be the public fuckup so everyone looking at me would say, "He's a fucking hellion. He's out of control." And that way whatever else was going on was ignored.

In that sense, my brother Bob and I had to have different experiences. Bob didn't know much of what was happening to me as a kid, between my dad and me. He couldn't and I didn't want him to, and that put distance between us. There was a leaving that took place when I was seventeen. My brother and I had come to a real parting of the ways. It was never anything hostile or resentful. It was kind. Bob was my father's public side and I was his private side, so separation between us seemed the right way to proceed. Bob has always been sweet-spirited and honorable in dealing with our separation, but it remained an unalterable fact for a long time. When he did finally learn what happened, with my father, and at camp, it just gave a name to everything.

* * *

There was another event that fundamentally shaped me around that time, and it had to do with my best friend Judgy. When you're young, if you're lucky, you encounter someone who sustains a compelling innocence. Judgy was a character right out of Fitzgerald. You always had the feeling of "be quick"—somehow it was an impermanent situation.

You'd have bet your bottom dollar that Judgy was touched by God. He'd greet me with "Milchy!" He had a pure appetite for experience. He wanted everything twice. We got into trouble when we were four and we stayed in trouble until we were about seventeen. Always raising hell. Always in the construction sites. We both had brothers. He had two—Torchy and Mark, both older. Torchy rode over my head with a bike once, and when I ran inside to ask my dad for help he just looked at me and said, "What? I'm shaving. You're fine."

When we were little we were on ball teams together. I didn't play baseball, I played at it. I liked it well enough, but Judgy was great. Gifted. We went to the same public elementary school and then the same private high school. I was a year older and they had skipped me a year from kindergarten to second (miserable), so we didn't have classes together. I'd see him in the halls. Judgy was a mess, and he wasn't a play-mess—he was a mess down to the ground. There was a recklessness in him that was oblivious to consequence.

Judgy's dad, Jim, was an alcoholic and an imponderable. You didn't know what the fuck he was going to do. We didn't want to make any mistakes with him, we just wanted to stay on this side of the ledger. If drinking with him was the price, then that's what we were going to do. Jim was a down-home alcoholic, no ifs, ands, or buts, unconflicted. His favorite expression was "People wonder why I fucking drink." Jim was looking for his excuses from the time he woke up, and if they weren't at hand he manufactured them. Jim, when he was in his cups, was always claiming the upper crust as his companions and consorts. "Oh Jesus Christ! Henry! I know *Henry*. God knows how many years . . ." Judgy's true given name was Almon. Almon Wheeler Lytle in full, but they all called him Judgy from the jump. Almon was his grandfather's name too and he was a state supreme court judge, so Judgy got the title as well. Judgy's Mom drank pretty good too. When she was drunk she'd take her teeth out, put them in water beside her 7-and-7.

Maybe the least attractive aspect of Jim's personality was the way his response to Judgy, his son, was instinctively to beat him. By way of testimony to not only evincing concern for Judgy, but also demonstrating a kind of moral superiority in himself by punishing him. Sounds not just a little bit like my own father. But Judgy and I didn't talk about that. And Jim took the fact that my dad halfway took him under his wing as proof of my dad's worthiness. We'd be drinking at his house and he'd grab me and say to me, "C'mere, c'mere. Now *Elmer— that's* a human being. That's an A-number-one, hundred-percent American human being. I'll give you a smack. Why don't I hang out with him? Because I have too much respect to be associated with him."

My father beat me differently. He always held one back, my dad. And in the one that he held back was an almost dramaturgical impulse to demonstrate his abstention from the deepest kind of hurt. Morally superior in his own way. Judgy and I were both aware that the other guy's father was treating him like that. Jim would lay a hand on me too, on occasion, or hit Judgy in front of me. There was a token quality to it. He wasn't looking to hurt, he was looking to dramatize. "You see this? You see this, Elmer Milch's kid? Watch this." *Smack.* "C'mere. You think you're done?" *Smack.* "C'mere." Judgy could only stand by because it wasn't real. It hurt twice as much for not being real. It was a demonstration of a kind of disrespect that Jim would use another kid as that kind of dramatic token.

I remember once, playing playground softball, we acted as if it were soft ground and we were ready to dive into it, to bruise ourselves, to slide. Jim was coaching Judgy and me. And Judgy makes a hit to right field through the hole between first and second, rounds on the way to second and slides. Tears his fucking leg right open. And Jim, by way of demonstrating his superiority to paternal flinching, comes down on Judgy twice as hard. "Oh, how bad is it? Maybe you better piss yourself." Jim would tell the story of what had happened afterward and Judgy hated it because he was pathologizing him and it wasn't really anything to be proud of, but that meant he had to go in with redoubled force. He cut the shit out of his leg. What was the point I was trying to make? I think it had to do with what Jim was showing, that he made no special call for his son. He dragged him up. "Why don't you piss yourself while you're at it?"

Two mean fathers.

The first time Judgy and I got drunk was together and I was probably eight and a half. I took the bottle from my parents, Black Label scotch. It was a bit intense and certainly we were sick. And who touted the event? Jim. "C'mere, kid. I want you to tell me the story of the last fifteen minutes. I'm so proud of you."

My father kept his distance from Jim, but he understood at some level that if he were to knock Jim down in Judgy's estimation, it would be a terrible sacrifice. Judgy liked my father. He loved to call him Elmer. It drove my father crazy. "It's Doctor

Milch." I loved Judgy for just that alone. It ought to have been beneath my dad to care about that. But he did.

If we got my dad in his well-oiled state, he'd grab Judgy and say, "We're going to talk for a few minutes now about the ways of the Jewish."

"Okay, mister."

"Yeah, call me mister again. I enjoy it."

"Doctor, I'm sorry."

"Jesus Christ."

My mother drank right before dinner, but nothing more than that. That was a road my dad walked alone.

We'd have to retrieve Jim from the bar sometimes and it was a bad scene. The bartender didn't want to have to kick him out, and he especially didn't want to do it in front of Judgy. The bartender didn't want to humiliate Jim in front of his kid, but he'd call us to come get him. So we'd go in and make up some reason we needed him, and Jim would leave with us and invariably posture, "This is very important, what you're doing. Very important. Don't let up. You've been thinking of a political career, haven't you? You may very well be in line. What are we talking about? A gubernatorial position? Who says no? Why are you denied the possibility that the next five guys we see shouldn't be denied?"

Judgy would sometimes take me to one side and he'd say, "David, this is very, very important: If by any combination of chances you wind up with a tongue in a strange pussy, do not weaken."

I want to say my first date was with Linda Chalmers. I used to have nightmares about her all the time. I'd be walking to school and I would elevate a little bit, just two feet off the ground, and she'd see me on the way and she'd tsk. "Dave." Tsk. "There goes Dave." Probably the genesis of levitation in

John from Cincinnati comes from that nightmare. Judgy and I tended not to trot our girlfriends out in front of each other, but a lot of times it happened. I want to say Judgy's first girlfriend was named Lois, but I know I'm wrong. If we fell in love, we didn't do it in front of each other. If we had, it would have been imposing a little bit upon him. *If it wasn't her, it'd be three others. What difference does it make?*

I lost my virginity to a hooker in Buffalo with Judgy. It's an inelegant story. Someone had the idea one day: "It's time." We were in a bar populated by not a few women of easy virtue of whom I picked one. I remember she had a teddy bear in her room upstairs. I came home with a shit-eating grin on my face and pulled my brother aside to tell him, "Guess what I did?" Before, I'd mostly gone to the Pine Grill for the music. There was a time when I was really into that. Judgy was into jazz too. Another night, we were seeing the Rhoda Scott Trio and Judgy said he'd be my best man if I proposed to Rhoda, so I did.

Graduation from high school I remember only in vague generalities. I was not the valedictorian. I filled out an application to both Harvard and Yale and my dad threw out the application to Harvard. There was a man named Inky Clark who recruited me to Yale, talked to my dad, and I think he had something to do with Dad's strong preference. My dad didn't talk to me about it. It was notable at that time for a Jew to go to Yale. You were made to feel they were giving you some special dispensation, that you were there by their favor. But when it was time I was ready to go.

Those first years, school breaks, my family would know I was coming home from college not because there had been any communication, but because a few boxes of dirty clothes would arrive the night before. My brother would pick me up at the train station and on one occasion I had about six migrant workers in tow. I had assured them of a hot meal. My folks did not react well. It disrupted routine. At the time, I was betting on sports and I'd been doing pretty well. Then I had a losing streak and instead of dropping back I pushed harder and lost more money than I ever thought I could lose. The bookie said, "They let you act like a man, then they turn you into a little boy again." I didn't tell my old man. I just hustled. I had enough problems.

Judgy was a hope-to-die alcoholic, but he didn't have anything to do with heroin. He'd be lying in his own puke and look at me and say, "How can you do that to your body?" I think I got introduced to it my last year in high school. I don't really remember the first time I tried it. I remember more the three or four hundred times I took it after that first time, and the effect was about the same.

Judgy started college at Cornell. I was reading at that time, but he wasn't particularly interested in that—he was still an athlete. I was into Dostoyevsky and Crane. While we were apart, I felt I was betraying something in that I undertook an openness to behavior that I should've undertaken with him. As much interest as I experienced while I was in school, there was always this pang of knowing I should've been there with Judgy.

Then Judgy died drunk in a car accident. He was with a fraternity brother of his, but different stories went around about who was actually driving. It wasn't even a tough road, they said, but if you're drunk enough, any road can be. He was a wonderful athlete and friend and a hope-to-die drunk and then he was dead for a fact. All unaware, Judgy had a native grace, it shone, and a hollowing ache came in realizing whatever organized the world could not sustain his presence. There was a terrible reality and finality in that—having been in the presence of a soul beautiful in its imperfections, then feeling it irretrievably gone.

My parents called to tell me he had died. They told me they had heard he died from another mother in town but that no one in Judgy's family had called, and didn't that say something. They tried to tell me to stay at school, not to come home, not to come back for the service. I said I was coming home. I remember staying drunk. I got drunk on the train back and then stayed that way the whole time. Good and drunk. But I can't generate the circumstances now. I know I was protective of it and didn't want to share my grief with anyone. I can remember being in an alley outside a bar and a vision of him came to me and he was trying to make me better than I was. "Hey, Milchy. What the fuck? What the fuck? Are you going to change your fucking underwear?" Trying to tease me out of a selfish remorse. Essentially saying, "Go out and be with me."

In many ways Judgy's death was a crossing of the river, eradicating everything you felt was impervious to change so you would be different for the rest of your life, and you realized with that seeping into you what it had meant to have been a child, what it was going to mean for life to be different forever. There was a pervasive sense of inauthenticity, that the fact on its own terms wasn't available to understanding. Our friends in their varied uncertainties and stumblings as they collected for his funeral and burial, unequal to the process of grieving "properly" but being of that process absolutely, registered a certain sheepishness, an admission that we had misunderstood everything about what life was. A truth was communicated when Judgy died. An unqualified fact that death was the organizing principle, and that truth either shaped your behavior or marked you as one who acts by turning away.

I remember we went to the racetrack, an act of defiance: We were going to do what we used to do and he wasn't going to be dead. We crossed the Peace Bridge into Canada and we started crying. Because Judgy had a gift that, if you're lucky, you experience in one person—an unalloyed joy about him—and when we went over the Peace Bridge we realized that he was gone for good and never coming back, the demarcation point between those who knew mortality as an idea and those who knew it in its fact. It was like we were six years old.

We picked up Jim, who was good and loaded, in a bar on the other side of the Peace Bridge. He'd already been kicked out of the house by then, a few months before Judgy died. In one of my last calls with Judgy we were talking about it, about what to do for Jim. Jim had sensed that there was something extraordinary in Judgy and he tried to articulate it. Finally he just asked me for twenty dollars, which was a truth of its own.

And you wonder why I drink.

I didn't stay in touch with the family or my friends after Judgy died, not more than once or twice, because we were illuminated as to the nature of reality in that moment and didn't want to be reminded of it. "If I hang out with them, I'm going to have to be thinking about that." Suddenly the solution to the problem was very clear: You don't hang out with them anymore.

But I didn't stop thinking about it. I thought about it even more, and that's what got me writing. I was ashamed that I had walked away from the experience. But I didn't really; I came back to it in a different way, and it was a liberation.

What I was writing became the start of a novel that I called *The Groundlings*, and that was my way of being with Judgy's family, writing about them in their grief. The groundlings was the name for the crowds in the cheap seats at Shakespeare's plays (which weren't seats, they had to stand). There's a quote in Melville's final work, *Billy Budd, Sailor*:

Passion, and passion in its profoundest, is not a thing demanding a palatial stage whereon to play its part. Down among the groundlings, among the beggars and rakers of the garbage, profound passion is enacted. And the circumstances that provoke it, however trivial or mean, are no measure of its power.

Each chapter of *The Groundlings* is with a different family member; they're never with one another, they're each alone with their grief. But I could be with them, and myself, in the writing in a way I couldn't otherwise. You'll see that stays true. It's easier for me to be fully present in my work than in my life. Here's how I wrote the call from my parents in that book, in the version I would turn in for my senior thesis:

Willy's parents had not wanted him to come home. His mother, who had placed the call to Willy that morning, had begun the conversation with a tearful plea that her son remain at school, that he could be no help to "him" now, that such affairs were inevitably morbid, that a heavy snowfall was expected. Willy had anxiously asked what was wrong, that he had made no plans to come home, and what was wrong. His mother had been silent for a moment, then had asked if Willy meant that those people had not even had the common decency, that after all the things, they had not even had the common decency to call him. Please, Willy had said, just please tell him what was going on. His mother had quietly observed that Willy had best speak with his father, she would go upstairs and pick up on the extension, and Willy's father could talk to him from down here.

His father had told Willy of Judge's death. He had said that he was not familiar with the details, they had only heard because Trish Wilcox had heard from her son at Cornell and had called Willy's mother, and had not been familiar with the details, but that as he understood the situation, Judge had been in an accident last evening, and that as he understood it the memorial service was to be held on Sunday, four days from now, including today. Willy had not replied. Willy must understand his mother's feelings in this situation, his father had continued, though he would leave it up to Willy, he was old enough now to make his own decisions, as to whether or not he should come home. All right, Willy had said distantly, he would see them at home. All he could do, his father had replied, was to try and give Willy the benefits of his own experience in this situation, to tell him that it had never been his own practice to go where he was neither needed or wanted. He would get a train, Willy had said, and see them at home. He had not been called, his father had replied, he could only try to remind Willy that he had not been called yet, and it was already ten in the morning. Did that tell him anything about how much he was needed or wanted by the Lytles? Did that remind him of anything certain parties had been telling him about the Lytles for some time now, about what kind of people they were. Willy had said he was coming home, he was coming home, and he would get a cab from the train station with the roads bad. Please leave it alone until he got home and they would discuss it. He would not stand in Willy's way, his father had answered. All he could say was his disappointment in this situation, but Willy was old enough now. There had followed a prolonged silence, broken by his mother's saying "Willy?" After another pause Willy had finally said, "I love you." "We love you too," his parents had replied in unison, and then had hung up the phone.

In the aftermath of Judgy's death, in the writing, some element of forgiveness registered. You were never going to be the same, had lived into the realization of your shortcomings, your inadequacies of spirit, and nothing was going to change that. Just the way it was, so you might as well try to learn to live with a little dignity.

I don't have a concept of God, but I feel as though there is some sort of pulsing thing. And the state of grace is for that thing to inhabit something else. I wish to hell I knew how to make that happen. I don't know how to enter that state as an act of volition; I just have to stay available. One thing you feel is that if you ain't there, it ain't coming. So I'm still in the process of finding out what His part is. For a long time the closest I came was after Judgy passed—I was able temporarily to re-create my connection with Judgy with words, with writing. It was a frightening experience but it was also elevating, such a fluid and maddening transaction. I felt the loss more acutely, feared pursuing it. You really only have a sense of the truth of that connection when you're in the midst of it.

After that it's gone.

2.

Strategies of Indirection

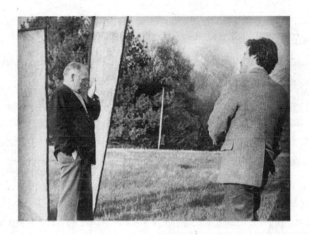

I FIRST MET ROBERT PENN WARREN as an undergraduate, because of my writing about Judgy. I had taken some classes with R. W. B. Lewis, a younger teacher and critic who in a way invented the discipline of American Studies as we know it now, and he read some of what I was writing and then contacted Mr. Warren and sent me over to him. Mr. Warren had already written *All the King's Men* by then, and won the Pulitzer for that novel and another one for his poetry. There was a paternal generosity in the way he carried himself and a kind of purity in his love for the material. You were always suppressing the impulse—"Is this guy kidding?"—because of his purity of spirit.

Lewis sends me to him but I'm still me so instead of just

going, first I follow Mr. Warren around for four days. Then I go to his door at dinnertime, knock, hand him a chapter, and ask him to read it right there. He just looked at me.

"Well, you act like a writer."

But he liked the work, and he told me so. He said, "No one writes dialogue better than you."

But that wasn't enough for me, so I said, "I don't know if I want to write anymore."

"Understand, David, I don't give a good goddamn who writes and who doesn't."

I had to know it was up to me.

James Joyce said paternity is not necessarily a matter of blood. I think that part of the journey of our spirits is to find our fathers. I remember my dad saying to me when I was knocking around in all kinds of trouble, "If you wanted to be a doctor, I could help you. Even if you wanted to be a thief, I could help you. But I can't help you with what you want to be. Someday you'll meet someone who can help you, and then it's your job to ask." With Mr. Warren, I asked.

The 150 pages of a novel I wrote were what I turned in for my senior thesis. I hadn't even been an English major before my senior year, so that was a turn of events. But I just kept writing the thing. You look at it now, it's almost all dialogue. What's not dialogue is nearly all description of physical action. To the extent that the physical world appears within it, it's in how people interact with it, stepping their foot in the snow, toeing a piece of garbage. I've never had too much interest in how things look beyond people. The exception was the final chapter, about Judgy's mom. That was a sort of stream-of-consciousness recounting of obsessive-compulsive behavior—scrubbing four times, things like that—repetitive phenomena that I could get caught in myself, that then becomes a kind of internal conversation with God. Mr. Warren liked that chapter. He thought it pointed to a way for me to write that wasn't so dependent on dialogue, even if dialogue was my strength. One of the other big critiques from more than one of the graders at Yale, including Mr. Warren, was that the symbolism of the names was too overwrought—"Judgy" (judgment), "Mark" (of Cain), "Torchy" (the light). I was too embarrassed to tell them those were just their real names.

I only took two classes with him as an undergraduate. There was so much to assimilate so quickly, and there was Mr. Warren in whom there was no self-division, at least no identifiable self-division, and you were almost embarrassed not to be a wholly unified soul in his presence. He was a gentleman, because that's what a man was supposed to be. The example of his identity was so much more powerful than his teaching. In certain respects, he wasn't a great teacher. But he so embodied a passionate involvement in the complexities of the material and manliness in such an unqualified fashion that everything else became subordinate. He would read poetry, just read it to us, and sometimes he would say, "Oh, isn't that fine." It was a small enough class that I felt he could see me and that I had better get to writing. He was a heroic person. "Be quick." I didn't know then that I'd get more time with him.

In college you start rehearsing the stories you're gonna tell about your family, about how you grew up. I talked about my dad a lot. Lots of medical knowledge coming from Dave, as if by osmosis. I'd diagnose anybody. My roommate Jeff Lewis, one thing he'd say later, the first thing he noticed about me was that I had "complicated and huge" feelings about my dad. I would tell stories about the Kefauver hearings—the Senate hearings in 1950 that showed most of the country the Mob was real. My dad would do surgeries for guys so they didn't have to testify. When I'd tell the story, the number of guys varied from my one uncle to dozens living in our house for weeks. My dad doing surgeries on dogs in our living room.

I joined a fraternity, Delta Kappa Epsilon—they thought my antics were fun. I was the token Jew. My friend Willie Monaghan was the token intellectual. Two of my friends were football players, Foster MacKenzie III and Bob Greenlee; Greenlee was the captain. They were musicians. We could get into some trouble, a lot of acid. We had motorcycles. I had a Norton 650. We'd go up by East Rock at night and play a game we called Random Particles. You close your eyes, open the bike as far as it'll go, and the first guy that opens his eyes is the loser. One time Bobby went right off the cliff. Bobby and Foster started a band called Prince La La and the Midnight Creepers, after the blues legend Prince La La—he died of a heroin overdose in 1963. They'd eventually become Root Boy Slim and the Sex Change Band. Foster was Root Boy and Bob played bass. Their biggest hit was "Boogie 'Til You Puke," which we did.

One weekend I went away for a wedding and during the course of the festivities I ended up duck hunting with my fraternity brother George W. Bush. There would eventually be an article published in *The New York Times* about the subculture of hazing within the fraternity system and some reporter had called our house to get statements, wanted to talk to George, who was president of DKE at the time. I answered and said, "Speaking." The reporter asked, "Could you confirm that you beat your pledges?" I told that reporter, "Not only do we beat 'em, we bugger 'em too!" When the article came out, George knew exactly who to come to. I liked him.

John Kerry was there then too. He was in the Pundits, which was like a highbrow comedy group of a kind. They invited me to one of their events and I got up at the end and retold each of the jokes they had already told, except that I made them funny. I don't know that John liked that approach.

I was there and I had friends and found my teachers, but I still had this voice in my head, "I'm not really like them. I'm a degenerate." And with my degenerate friends maybe I told myself, "Well, I don't quite fit in here either, do I? I'm supposed to be reading." Now looking back, clearly I was a part of all of it. I'm not this or I'm not that, that was the lie. But you don't feel that at the time.

Floyd was the acid manufacturer on campus. I can't remember which of Robert Penn Warren's poems has the line "The filth of self, to be loved, must be clad in glory." That was Floyd. He wore a cape and a stupid tall hat. He was making money, but he didn't come from it. He found me. I was famously loaded and I think I was still in the flirtation phase with smack. I wasn't shooting, I was snorting. There was a profound line between shooting and snorting. Floyd came looking because he wanted to cop heroin, to make a trade.

I remember driving a car into the ocean, but I don't remember the associated events. There was a house in Milford, Connecticut. I was on acid. About seven people lived there, not me. People were constantly in transit. I think I was still an undergraduate. I wouldn't swear to all of this, but the car and the water I know. The cops didn't find the trunkful of weed and when the police finally left, the friend I was with said, "Dave, I know that was a lot of fun for you, but it was all drag for me."

Because I'd been on a bender with a bunch of fraternity brothers, my graduation weekend at Yale found me intensely hungover. My father had decided I was continuing on to Yale Law. The way he put it was, "When I was your age, I wanted to go to law school"—the jabbed finger being the exclamation point on "and that's what you're going to do!" His family had delivered a similar edict when my old man graduated, except the specifics had been medicine, and so the cycle looped around. When my eldest was eight years old, I said to her, "I've been holding this back as long as I could. I want you to go to Yale." I like to tell myself she still felt it was her choice. Those edicts are their own expression of love, however distorted or distorting.

Dad had done his undergraduate work at the University of Buffalo. He was proud of me at the graduation. Hungover himself but feeling accomplished. There was a hotel one block over from the Taft and closer to campus, where my mom and dad both stayed that weekend. He was in a sheer alcoholic blizzard. Strong that way. He would get meaner or nicer on the bottle depending on the way the wind blew. If someone rubbed him the wrong way, he'd get ill-tempered. But if they were pleasant or good-natured he'd lean into it. He liked to impress my friends, particularly my Gentile friends. He would confide to lampposts if no one else was available: "When I was your vintage I was blind drunk every day I drew breath." But there was nothing malicious about him toward my friends. They were intimidated by him nonetheless, but his being loaded neutralized whatever might have been imposing or off-putting. He was a great one for placing his hand on the other person's wrist to explain a crucially important point having to do with nothing whatsoever. It was a pleasure to see him relax. My father would gesture toward the campus at large: "Now this is a different version of the same fucking thing. You keep your nose down, you make a good fucking living. You want to make a mistake at night, nobody's gonna hold that against you."

Upon graduating in 1966 I was awarded the Chauncey Brewster Tinker Prize, baby. It's a prize in English. I was actually short the credits I was supposed to have for the major since I had come to it late. They had comprehensive exams in those days and almost didn't let me take the test, but they consented and then I got the highest marks in the history of the exam. Neither I nor my parents seemed interested in the implications of that. I had no idea if I was covering up my drunkenness in front of them. I went off with friends afterward. I think we went up to Poughkeepsie, to Vassar. I had to make a port of call there.

* * *

The truth is the timeline from 1966 to 1970 is pretty confusing, nationally as well as personally, but my being loaded then and losing my mind now doesn't help trying to reconstruct it. Mr. Warren and Dick Lewis were on one side, trying to help me write, and my dad was on the other, trying to get me to law school.

I sold the novel and got an advance to finish it. I may have sold it more than once, to get more than one advance. Lillian Hellman liked my work and took me to a few parties. Thanks to Mr. Warren and Mr. Lewis, I did a first round at the Iowa Writers' Workshop in '67.

That was a time when everything was upside down. Bad habits were fostered. I wasn't a dilettante. I wasn't doing drugs because I thought they made my work more interesting. It was for real. I did a little writing in Iowa, kept working on *The Groundlings* about Judgy. I started adapting the five chapters of the novel I'd written as an undergraduate into a play. I made a friend named Michael Ruggere who was in the drama program. He also liked heroin. We performed *The Groundlings* there. I played Jim and Michael directed. My attendance was sporadic, but I was good and fucked up so when I showed up, my presence was noticed. When I was attending, I lived in the Hotel Jefferson. I had an apartment, but I could never get there. I was always too ripped. That was where the bifurcation came into play—to be able to do both. I was lucid, but I spoke very slowly. If I was feeling pain about Judgy dying or anything else, I was making sure I didn't. I was a jerk in seminars. I'd tear other students' work apart. Kurt Vonnegut and Richard Yates were teaching there then, and they both hated me. They were self-taught and proud of that, unfinished in their own way. They drank as much as I did, but coming from Yale, on Mr. Warren's word, I was everything they hated. In the Yates biography by Blake Bailey, there's a story about a night at Kenney's Bar when Richard laid into me, "Who wouldn't want to be David Milch? He went to Yale! He graduated first in his class! Warren said he has an ear for dialogue that rivals Hemingway! And here he is *twenty-one years old*. . . ." He saw it all as pretension, and he wasn't wrong.

I was at Iowa for a year of the two-year program. While I was there, I got involved with this acid-manufacturing project, so I went to Mexico and was making acid (rather well, I might add). When I came back up to Iowa City they had bought a farm and set up a laboratory, so I helped with that, which wasn't the standard course of the writers' program.

My role at the lab was to get through the day, one day at a time. There was a lot of money to be made. There were a lot of guns. Several people expired. Not by my hand, but they were sufficiently proximate to give me hard pause. I didn't kill them, but I might as well have. I was using acid at the time, but didn't stop there. Tire sealer. Tire sealer is a much undervalued commodity. I remember bouts of mania, bouts of depression. Lots of heroin mixed in there. The hallucinogens gradually lost their appeal. Heroin wasn't attractive, but it felt good. Never underestimate the simple thing.

I remember once I buried myself in Mexico and that got my attention. I was working for these criminals, that would be the fair way to put it. I had gotten involved by steps. I'd sold my passport to a guy about six months before, and at the time I'd told myself, "And that's as far as I go!" Six months later I'm down in Mexico doing the rest of this stuff and there's a chemist down there, this lunatic chemist—bottle glasses, he'd get into a car and he'd have an accident within two hundred feet. He would hit a burro or something and start throwing pesos everywhere. He contracted a bit of a stomachache, and he had a consort named Yum-Yum who decided to treat his stomachache with an enema.

As it turned out he had peritonitis and she killed him with this enema. We were all down there illegally and so I'm out there digging this guy's grave. We're tossing the body in there and now I think, "Well, let me see if I can get some ID in case at some point I try to do the right thing and contact his relatives and let them know the news of his finish." I take out his ID and it was me. He had my passport that I had sold six months before. So that gave me some pause. And only the most liberal applications of chloroform kept that moment of clarity from extending into a protracted bout of lucidity and perhaps a life change, but that's why they make chloroform, and I was able to keep going for a number.

That was Cuernavaca.

Then we were in Redlands. Then Berkeley. Then the farm. I should have been afraid I'd die. I was certainly doing everything possible to be eligible. But somehow I made it through.

After however many months of that, in Iowa's mind I wasn't really enrolled anymore, so my dad prevailed and I started Yale Law School. I think in those days you just signed your name to a list. But I felt somewhat ambivalent about attending, as evidenced by a letter from that time:

> To John, Elaine, and Tuck
> Very brief, to let you know I am alive and well, in law
> school at Yale for a duration yet to be determined. Still
> trying to write, always drunk, the same old songs. Write
> and will start correspondence with whole sentences and
> paragraphs. Vin is assistant commissioner of small parks in
> NYC and Jeff is at Howard Law. I can go no further.
>   Love,
>   David

I remember some, but I was loaded sunrise to sunrise. Wake up and not know where I was, which isn't recommended for law students. You know when you're dreaming and you've missed a class for the whole year and all of a sudden you have to sit for the exam? I went back and lived this dream. Most days I couldn't even get to the school. There was one day I actually went and took an exam in one of my classes because I was loaded and figured it'd be kind of fun. Torts. Afterward, I see the teacher, who actually went on to—I don't know what he became, a pretty important justice or something. But he looks at me and takes a huge breath and he says, "You don't even know what a tort *is*, do you?" I just walked away.

I hated it so bad. I hated even just the thought of it. I never got any books or anything. At that time, the credit card companies, in a policy they have since reconsidered, used to send out free credit cards because you're a college graduate. So I have this massive credit card, and I'm living in a hotel—I think it was the New Haven Inn out by the Wilbur Cross Parkway. The months are going by, and finally I go up to my room at the school. It's like two months after class is in session, and for the first time, I go up to my room. This kid is there, this dick from Brandeis, and I'm all fucked up, and he says, "Oh, I've heard so much about you, and you know, they said you're completely unstable."

"Well, you know, yeah, I got some problems, I mean."

"When you go to class, what kind of notebook do you write on?"

"Well, I haven't been to class."

"Yellow? White? Do you have, like, these three-ring, do you use the loose leaf?"

Now, I know all the furniture in the room is his because I don't have any furniture. I say, "Steve, I want you to watch me for the next five minutes. Let me break your furniture."

"That's what they said, you were crazy. I'm a little scared. I want to be honest with you, you're frightening me a little bit."

"Let me frighten you."

I throw some of his clothes out the window and I leave.

*   *   *

One particular night I found myself shooting up traffic lights with a shotgun. I believed that when I fired the gun, I could make the lights change color. I might have taken the shotgun from one of the masters' houses at Yale, or that might have been a sword from a different incident. Or, now that I think about it, maybe I had the sword and then I found the shotgun and so I made a switch. It happened that I was on acid at the time. I failed to notice the very different nature between traffic lights and police lights, and so I began shooting at the police lights too. At some level it occurred to me that this was mistaken behavior. So I picked up some shotgun shells and ran up to the officers and said, "Some guy is shooting up the place! He's out of his mind!" The police said, "Yeah, we know. We got it." And like an idiot, I just sat down. I had been arrested before. I was known to the police in New Haven. When the cop came up to me, I said, "I'll confess when your badge stops melting."

The dean of the law school said, "I can't keep you in, Milch." I said, "I wouldn't keep me either." And that was it. How about that for being white? You can shoot at a cop car and get sent to the law school dean. I may have even been aware of that incongruity at the time, but the truth is more that I thought the world revolved around me. The other upside was I was deemed ineligible for the draft, which in my mind had been the primary virtue of law school to begin with.

I'm going in circles. I promise you: What it feels like now reading it is only a fraction of the confusion it felt to be living it. Thanks to some generous advocacy, they let me back into Iowa.

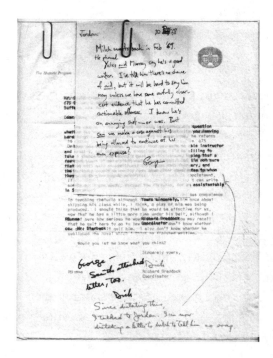

Gratitude and shame and entitlement all operating at varying levels each day. I graduated from Iowa in May of 1970. This time, I made it through with some success.

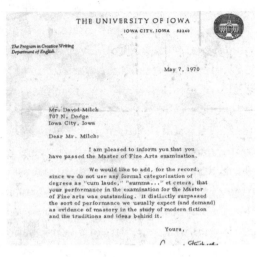

I had knowingly addicted myself to heroin because it provided structure. For me, using drugs was a way to organize and structure a day. I loved heroin. I loved checking out. You were here and you were not here at the same time. That has appeal. The thing with acid was that it was a mixed message. You were doubled up. You were loaded and you were transcendent, but with dope you were just loaded, which is all I ever wanted to be.

* * *

About six weeks after my graduation from Iowa, Mr. Warren and Mr. Lewis invited me to come back to Yale to teach and help them put together a literature textbook—*American Literature: The Makers and the Making*—along with another teacher and critic named Cleanth Brooks. Mr. Warren was very generous about it: "I will trust that this foolishness is at an end." There was something so brazenly stupid about my behavior that some small part of him couldn't help but be, I won't say amused, but amazed or something. Boy, I had to be lucky. There were a lot of left turns that could've been taken.

It was pretty clear it was time to fish or cut bait. I was going to have to become available to their disciplines and ambitions or there would be no collaboration. Preparing that textbook, encountering with the professors the work of those writers was a particular sort of joy, how given my teachers were to their undertaking, almost exalted. Sometimes you may see a horse ready to run in a race and the animal is so much itself in what it's about to do you feel privileged to be in its presence. We read everything, and they saw it all in conversation. Working on those materials, over years, you had to understand and incorporate into the fiber of your being that you were working in a tradition, that your work was part of a conversation with everybody. That became the air that we breathed.

The three professors sensed in me a self-division but they sufficiently respected the effort I was making to behave honorably, generate the work I was to do, never showing up obviously loaded, that the subject wasn't exposed. There were still tells. I never had a proper winter coat, would walk around New Haven in the dead of winter in a sports jacket. I lost my keys a lot, or maybe never had them to begin with, but my teachers brought me in from the cold.

The class I taught most in those years was called Strategies of Indirection in Fiction. This was the initial course description:

STRATEGIES OF INDIRECTION IN FICTION

The purpose of the course is to identify and study the various techniques by which the writer of fiction can gain access to the imagination of his reader, and thus can persuade the reader to stand in a given relation (i.e., the desirable relation) to the action of the work. It will be suggested that these techniques rely on the imaginative channelling of the reader's energies -- as against the logical demand upon those energies which one might notice in a different kind of prose writing. The process involves providing certain receptacles within the dramatic framework (a character, a new scene, a symbolic object) for emotional concerns which have been purposefully excluded by the narrative voice.

The process in fact, it will be argued, is double, and a parallel inquiry will be made into the vital source of these channelling techniques in the artist's attempt to circumvent the disciplines of his own consciousness. This he does not by suppressing his consciousness (as certain fashionable contemporary novelists seem to be trying to do), but by restricting it to the level of organization -- and, again, by deflecting his deepest emotional concerns to the action itself, or the true subject of his work.

In Moby-Dick, to take a supreme example, Melville can be seen, in the chapter on cetology, wilfully exhausting his rational consciousness as an instrument for "compassing" the whale, to the point where he can then project himself into Ahab's monomania. Simultaneously, those same chapters end by convincing the reader that cetology has nothing to do with the real nature of the white whale and of the action, as Ahab has all along been declaring.

It will perhaps be obvious that the critical perspective of this course has more in common with the methods of Kenneth Burke and, though much less so, with those of Wayne Booth than with the more familiar "craft of fiction" approach.

Examples of illuminating failure of the double process (e.g., Stone's Hall of Mirrors and the work of Robbe-Grillet) will be studied, along with some great successes.

Two papers, critical or creative, will be required.

The reading list will include:

Melville:	Moby Dick
	The Confidence Man
James:	The Wings of the Dove
Mann:	The Confessions of Felix Krull
Hesse:	Narcissus and Goldmund
Stone:	A Hall of Mirrors
Gardiner:	Fat City
Burke, K:	Selected Essays

What I was trying to teach was the idea that the reader or audience's experience of a work, how they feel as they go through it, is what conveys the work's argument, and that experience is usually different from the actual words. Another way of saying it is that form shapes content. With *Moby-Dick,* your faculties of understanding are exhausted by the work itself, and it's by having your faculties totally and utterly exhausted that you can feel Ahab's obsession with the whale and Ishmael's obsession with the story. "I'm taking it all in and I'm overwhelmed and I'm still not sure exactly what it means." That's what it means. Henry James uses a different tactic—he introduces a new character to a world and then through that character's misapprehension the reader comes to apprehend the world more clearly.

This was a writing class, but I went into it through reading. It's too much for a young student to constantly be looking at their or their classmates' work. If you bring something already taken for granted as literature and you workshop that, then we can have some fun. To suggest that our greatest writers might have been struggling with the same feelings, which we know for a fact they were, is a good thing for a writer to live into. There are ways to turn problems of spirit into problems of technique—that's another kind of indirection. Kafka was just a miserable, miserable human being. Pathologically shy and physically ill, but he wanted to tell stories. So one morning Gregor Samsa woke up and discovered he was a bug. All of his misery is now a problem of technique. How does a bug live in a family where the rest are human beings? People speak of the symbolic philosophical resonance of that work, but that is a domestic comedy.

There's something about literature—poetry and prose, but particularly poetry—which disinfects the effort of being. The effort itself is cleansing. It neutralizes what's profane about the process, and just leaves the result. That was always true about Mr. Warren's work, his essays and especially his poetry. There was an unapologetic elegance, a purity of purpose. He was like that as a person. Except, at another level, he was a country boy, which is how he grew up. But his commitment to the process of art purified everything that might have been considered other than pure. He just wrestled with the material unapologetically, until it seemed right, in a fierce commitment to it.

Mr. Warren was full of strength and generosity and was willing to believe the best of somebody until he was proven mistaken, and then to believe it again. He was disciplined in terms of what he would allow to be in play, what variables he would allow to shape the contours of the discussion; by his adhering to those high standards of discourse, you either did the same or you sort of ruled yourself out. His favorite expression in regard to me was always, "Well, how much of a goddamn fool can you be?"

Prior to Mr. Warren's teachings, I thought of the whole idea of poetry as unmanly. My dad had a profoundly skeptical attitude in that regard. That was one of the gifts Mr. Warren gave me: the neutralizing of that fastidiousness, the recognition of poetry as not only honorable but manly. And it was as if an entire shell fell away. One can, later, encounter one's childhood in an entirely different way. And Mr. Warren's unconflicted embracing of all of those emotional states was such a liberation. You know a lot of times when you're ten or twelve and there's a group of guys and there's one guy who's the leader of the pack, and it becomes unmanly to be other than "in his train"? That was what it was like to encounter poetry through Mr. Warren. It would have been unmanly, unhuman, to not get in his train.

I would get to go to Mr. Warren's house in Vermont when we were working on that book. I would stay in Shack Two, and we would work during the morning on the textbook, then early afternoons were saved for his poetry, and then late in the afternoon we would take long walks. That was a terrific time. Mr. Warren would also swim, but he took his swimming very seriously and he wasn't looking for companions. With poetry, his feeling was that one composes with one's whole being, physically too. His poetry was all unified. It was a process of breathing and training that would happen to him in the water.

Mr. Warren and I didn't talk about women, but we talked about work all the time. One of the liberations of my teachers' approach was the idea that everything you needed to understand a piece of art was in the work itself—that if you paid attention, the work would teach you its meaning through its form. That was the main idea of the so-called New Criticism. That's not to say that certain historical or biographical or philosophical ideas aren't relevant, but that if the work's good, the argument or themes are going to come through whether you know that other stuff or not. Mr. Warren would say, "Now go back and look at that again." He would have me read his commentaries on various literary figures we were anthologizing.

"Write two paragraphs on that."

A whole kind of animation would come over him when he talked about other writers' work or his own. It was extraordinary how alive the process was to him—how alive these writers, some dead for centuries, were in his imagination. His encounter with them was vital. They were alive and their work was alive and he was sitting with them. That was the kind of immediacy his conversation with their work generated: It was as if they were sitting there.

Mr. Brooks was a very different type of guy. Wore his Christianity as a kind of armor. He was very fastidious, brilliant, idolized Mr. Warren, but he carried his own water. They wrote a lot of books together, and Mr. Brooks did his share.

R. W. B. Lewis had the demonic in him. He's the only one I ever called by his first name. He was about ten years junior to Mr. Warren and Mr. Brooks, but I think it was because we shared an office. Dick was a drinker. I was forever bumping into him in compromising situations. He was the worst liar I've ever met. He would always say, "This is all very explicable." There were these dry moats around the colleges and so I would jump into the moat and climb in through the window because I didn't have my key, and he's the only guy who could have put up with that. He seemed to understand it perfectly. His friendship and advocacy could sometimes take on a gleeful extremity. After my first year teaching, in his course evaluation, he wrote: "I should also say, perhaps, that in addition to being intellectually stimulating in the highest degree, Milch is also a force for good in the college community—as a resolute, articulate, and persuasive opponent of all but the most harmless drugs, as a living example of youthful devotion to the humanistic arts, as a person of radical convictions who is also a firm believer in humane and civil behavior." He was trying to make somebody laugh, maybe just himself. To see me more or less surviving, or at least soldiering on, and watching all of my fallibilities play themselves out—I think Dick enjoyed that. The three of them were so different in the way they comported themselves personally, and that too was part of the lesson: It canceled out any thought that there was any one way.

It was so important to Mr. Warren to be honorable as a man, and the fact of someone like Theodore Dreiser's excellence as a writer cohabitating with the profundity of his being a shitheel always used to engage Mr. Warren. It was a paradox that in some sense was in conflict with his idea of the purifying resources of art. Secretly I think he was haunted by what he knew to be an illusion—that if you wrote well, there was some sort of purity in the activity of your imagination. He knew that to be true, but he knew as well without any doubt at all that the excellence of your work did not speak one way or another for your deportment as a man and it confounded him. He believed in the purifying capacity of art, even as he saw it refuted all around him.

My book stalled. I went through a six-month period where every day I rewrote the same twelve pages almost word for word. They were the pages in which Judgy's mom falls into obsessive-compulsive behavior. My publishing contract lapsed. I knew I had to get out of the loop, but even when I tried, other compulsions waited. Here's a PPS I wrote to Mr. Warren in 1974 from the writers' retreat at Yaddo, which he and Dick Lewis had gotten me into:

Last Saturday night, after a hard week's work and an hour's soul-searching, I decided to go to the racing track. As I came downstairs I saw, through the Tiffany window, a bolt of lightning. This was followed in short order by a serious clap of thunder. When I got outside I found that a tree limb had fallen on my car, and shattered the windshield. Can it be that God is this strict?

* * *

My office with Dick Lewis and my classes were all in what was then called Calhoun College. (I had been in Trumbull as an undergraduate. One of the worst things Yale does to you is make you feel compelled to identify your residential college at every opportunity for the rest of your life, even as you know there is not a single person on the planet who could give a fuck.) I often had money on football games and I let some of the students come watch at my apartment. One of the students was a kid named Gardy. One day when he was a junior we were talking in the courtyard and he introduced me to his younger sister Rita, who was then a freshman. She was in what was only the fourth class of women to attend all four years. Rita's sophomore year, I did a seminar with Dick Lewis that she took. We would see each other around campus.

I was dating a woman named Becky then. Premed, Gentile. We would eat dinner every night at a restaurant called the Old Heidelberg, because all that routine stuff I described about my old man not surprisingly became true of me too. Perhaps Rita noticed that routine or maybe the restaurant was just on her way home, but she would often pass by while we were eating. I don't think I picked up on all the possible implications of that, but Becky sure did. One dinner, she'd tell me that Rita slept with every man on campus. Another time, she said Rita had every part of her body operated on. Neither of these were true, but they did have the effect of allocating to Rita more of my attention.

I asked her to dinner for the first time just before Thanksgiving of her senior year in 1976, but she was busy so we didn't have the dinner until the next week. I flew her to Los Angeles to go to the races at Santa Anita that winter break. By February I took her to meet my parents in Florida and proposed. She was the first Jewish girl I'd ever dated and my father was dying. She was a German Jew, which barely counts, but my parents were still happy.

Rita was a fine arts major, a painter. Layers of collage and color. Third-generation Yale on her dad's side, which tells you just how thoroughly assimilated they were, and her mom's side was well-off too. Her mom had been seventeen when they married, and then they split up when Rita was fourteen, which was ahead of its time in its own way. Her mom didn't give a shit about Yale, even though all three of her kids went there.

Rita and I went to Chicago on the way back from Florida to tell her family we were engaged and Rita's mother was less thrilled. I was ten years older than Rita, and Jill, Rita's mother, was only twelve years older than me. I insisted on talking to her alone. She was lying on her bed and I sat on a bench across from her. I told her I was a drug addict who kept methadone in her daughter's refrigerator, and I showed her a scar on my leg that I said was from a gunshot (it sure looks like one, but I don't remember what happened). *You think I'm a jerk? I'll show you.* Somehow this didn't make her any more excited about the prospect of our marriage.

After we talked, I told Rita I'd never been so insulted in my life and that she would leave with me or we were finished. Later she would admit that her mother had offered to send her to Europe for a year to get her away from me, said I was a Svengali. But Rita came with me.

The Milford Jai Alai opened that spring, and with a new gambling institution opening just down I-95, I feel compelled to go. I take Rita, her friend Felicity, and a young local friend of mine named Oscar who'd just gotten out of jail. I think I'd maybe done a prison writing program with him. Rita and Felicity start making two-dollar bets. I'm with Oscar, getting into the odds, trying to cover every betting outcome, and I'm fucking losing. I go to check in on Rita and Felicity, and they tell me they've won. They're excited, happy, like college seniors a month from graduation having some fun, which is what they are. But that offends me. They're winning two-dollar bets. They don't know the fucking game, they're enjoying themselves. I'm pissed off and only half trying not to show it. At ten P.M. I say, "Let's get out of here." It had been light when we went in, but it's dark when we come out, and that's when I notice there's still some construction going on, the lights in the parking lot aren't hooked up yet. Now I start thinking out loud, "You know, this isn't very safe. You could be walking out with big winnings, cash in hand, and it's very dark out here and someone could be waiting and you wouldn't see 'em. They would be liable, with the lights not on yet. You could make a lot of money." We'd gotten in my Skylark at this point and Rita's next to me in the front seat and Oscar and Felicity are in the back. I turn around and say, "Oscar, hit me."

"What do you mean, Dave?"

"I'm gonna go back in and say I was robbed."

"No, Dave, I can't do that."

"Oscar! Come on. Hit me!"

"I just got out, Dave."

"Come on, Oscar!"

Finally he punches me in the face. It's an awkward angle so I really only get a bruise by my eye.

"Okay, let's go back in."

Now they're all scared, but they start following me back into the fronton because they don't want to piss me off even more. We're about to go inside, and some aspect of the situation hits me, maybe the risk I was putting Oscar to, and I stop. "Fuck it. Let's go home."

The next day another one of my friends went back and followed through and won a very nice settlement.

By that summer we were having dinners with Mr. Warren, Mr. Brooks, Dick Lewis, and their wives. Rita had graduated and we were still in New Haven. Perhaps some of the downsides of the overall situation were dawning on her. She had lost a lot of weight. She was drinking gin and tonics out of empty sour cream containers. On some level I noticed those things. She wanted to leave New Haven and I think it had become clear to her I wasn't going anywhere. We were on our way to the movies and she turned to me.

"I can't do this."

"Go to the movie?"

"No. This."

"Where should I drop you off?"

She drove to Chicago that night, then to Los Angeles for a job editing a horror movie. By Thanksgiving I visited and we got back together. She moved back to New York, worked on more movies, and I'd commute between there and New Haven. Rita would cut the film with scissors and fuse it back together. She worked on a documentary about the Sex Pistols that had the original Sid and Nancy footage at the Chelsea Hotel. I'd go visit her in the editing room and we'd talk about how to make that footage tell that story. We worked together with the music professor Willie Ruff on a documentary with Dizzy Gillespie. There would be more breaks along the way, a lot of living apart even when we were together.

The thing you must understand is that at every stage of Rita's and my courtship, and throughout our subsequent life together, I thought I would die fairly soon. When you believe that, you're willing to accept pretty much any outcome, because what difference could it make? But Rita was willing to believe a life was possible for us, and for me. That kind of belief is its own act of creation.

It was in this period, when Rita and I were long distance but our relationship was taking on a certain fixedness, that my work with my teachers began to shift from the textbook to other forms. My teachers made the people we studied so alive that soon enough I was imagining them up and about, and talking.

* * *

We read and discussed so many great writers during that period, but there was one family of writers who held particular sway over the professors and our work at the time and went on to have a profound effect on me, and that was the James family. In particular, three of the children: William, Henry, and Alice. They would be the subject of the first television show I ever conceived of—*The James Family*.

Dick Lewis was interested in the idea of the family and Mr. Warren much more so with the idea of William, and I was sort of ricocheting around among all those things, and I guess willy-nilly it came to be that my ricocheting became an organizing principle that framed the dynamic of the family's literary connections each with the others.

What we encountered when we looked at their lives and

their work was that the whole of the genteel tradition in America had been broken in two very different ways by two men who happened to be brothers—William James and Henry James. In order to understand this and them, we went back. The names repeat in different generations so prepare yourself. The first William James, William Sr., who helped build the Erie Canal and made a fortune in real estate and moneylending in the towns all along it, had twelve children. One of his children, Henry James Sr., suffered a terrible, terrible accident and lost his leg in a fire. His tutor, who failed to get him out of the fire, was Joseph Henry; years later he would help found the Smithsonian Institution. It struck us how such a vital institution that was responsive to new possibilities could have been created out of a series of accidents and duplicities. As to the hold of genteel tradition on American thinking, the first William James, the grandfather, was a Calvinist and he believed that the extent to which he was successful in business reflected God's judgment upon him. That's the secret suspicion of every asshole in Newport, Rhode Island—the faith that our family has been blessed because we should be blessed because we are whoever we are. But there was something so grotesque in the first William James invoking this idea, because he was such a prick and such a violent man. So here's this guy who, to make the world testify to the fact that God approves of him, underwrites the world around him, and becomes a trustee at his local Presbyterian church. He doesn't believe a goddamn thing, but he wants to buy the clerics to tell him that his work has been blessed, and everyone goes for it, except his own children. He broke every one of the kids, not one of them was worth a damn, except for his son Henry, the first Henry, whose wound as an amputee protected him. The first Henry couldn't be a man, so his father, the first William, didn't have to break him. He'd already lost his leg, so they let him read. And he read and read and read. He was verbally very rebellious. He didn't have a lot of experience, and he didn't understand the way that people took what he said, and so he was accused of being a lot of things when in fact he wasn't—he just didn't have the objective correlative. He read and he read and he read, and he didn't live a goddamn day in his life. He would take these idiotic tours of Europe, as a way for his father to wash his hands of him. But in that way, he never had inflicted upon him the structures that he needed to justify the fact that he was wealthy. He inherited a tremendous amount of money and never worked a day in his life, so he had no pieties about American business. No one taught him to be ashamed, so he was hospitable to every idea.

When he married, his occupation became the raising of his children, and he took them around Europe and never stayed still because he was always afraid that something was gaining on him. He would not let them embrace any single belief. They took in all the data of tradition with none of its structure. They had the perfect doubleness for the arts, to be inside and outside. All his efforts went toward the creation of these geniuses: Alice, William, and Henry.

There was no place for Alice James in the world beyond the family dynamic. She was first given to her brother William to mind, and she got sick. She found in dying her career, her occupation, and her love. Katharine Peabody Loring became her nurse, and they were able to accommodate all their feelings toward each other in this relationship. After the parents died, Alice went over to live with Henry in England and everyone came to call upon her. The journal that she began to keep when she was dying was absolutely extraordinary. It's beautiful and gossipy and just what you want. What she could have been, had the time allowed her, is a question for a different time. But for now, the art, the historical accident that changed American culture, came from her and the family accepting that William was "the guy."

There was no one who didn't love her brother William James. Her brother Henry was very shy and very much content to be in William's shadow, apparently. William was the one who was going to be out in the world and engaged, and Henry was going to be an observer. William went to Harvard and was going to be the great man of that class.

William James was a vigorous, sweet-spirited, healthy-minded guy. He was so charming and engaging and brilliant, everybody knew he was going to be an ace. William's problem was that he had no way to stand. His father had given him all of the data of experience and the blessing of saying, "You don't know what it means yet, but just take it." But to the structure of his life, he was no less an amputee than his dad was. He didn't know what the hell to do and so he took to his bed and became afflicted with terrible headaches and backaches and so on. Everybody began to whisper about poor William James—he had such a great future and he turned out to be a reclusive dick.

He had a teacher, Louis Agassiz, a great naturalist and mad man who documented all of Darwin's theories and was collecting specimens while refusing to believe in Darwin—he also insisted on being an unabashed racist. He came to the James house. William by this time was a physician who never practiced, but Agassiz came to the Jameses and he said, "William, we're going up the Amazon, we're collecting specimens." William said, "I can't get out of bed, let alone go up the Amazon." Agassiz answered, "I didn't ask if you can get out of bed."

Agassiz put him on the ship and took him up the Amazon and literally threw him off the boat. And in that moment was born every aspect of William James's philosophy, which is that you cannot think your way to right action, you have to act your way to right thinking. And from that came the James idea of pragmatism, that the good is what works, and that we rewire ourselves by our behavior.

This allowed William James to figure out that you don't have to integrate the American experience into any preexisting structure, it is an unfolding. Accept it as such. Don't try to put names on it. That was a refutation of the whole exhausted rationale of gentility. "It's good because we've always done it that way." What James said was, "Who cares how you've always done it, just how are you doing it, how does it work?" And that brought all American behavior into the sunlight of thought. Because otherwise what you are saying is everything is invincibly vulgar, it's impossible and we must have nothing to do with it. There had developed in America a practice among the gentility of flinching from public life because it was so vulgar, and here was William James throwing open the goddamn doors and saying it's all in play.

Henry, in his way, was standing outside, but he was hospitable to every story being available as material for rendering, to every aspect of the American story.

The example of these two men—of one or the other of these two men—has been followed by nearly every figure who has contributed to American culture ever since. Through everyone that William taught—and he taught everybody, including Gertrude Stein—and everyone who knew and read Henry.

You could see all of America in them and they were such full people and it could have been a great show. Dick Lewis and I pitched it together to the National Endowment and PBS and all those places. I was writing scripts and he was writing a book—the book he would actually publish. In 1979, we were down at the National Endowment getting dough, and Dick was called out of the room while we were pitching.

We finished and afterward we went out and had some coffee. I said, "I think that went pretty well." We were talking the meeting through and about ten minutes in he said, "Listen, when I was called out of the room, they were telling me that your father had died, taken his life, and his instructions were that you were not to be told until after the pitch was finished."

My dad had been sick for a while with stomach cancer, and my brother, who idolized my dad the same way I did, had taken over my father's care. My dad would engage in self-mutilation and all sorts of unpleasant things, and in his tormented mind, because his sense of self was so associated with his professional identity as a physician, he became convinced that since my brother had become the caregiver in the family, my brother was having sexual relations with my mother. He took his life in front of them, to punish them for that, and then his last words were, "Don't tell David until he's done with his pitch."

Or at least that's how I've remembered it. Bob would get quiet whenever it came up.

* * *

I kept working, like my dad wanted me to. I kept fucking up, like my dad wanted me to. When I wrote to Mr. Warren to tell him my father had passed, I started by congratulating him for his latest Pulitzer. "I write also to tell you that the long cruelty of my dad's illness ended last month. My parents' love survived all the illness's indignities and my mother seems able—if somewhat tentatively—to look to the future." The letter ends with me asking if I could come visit. I just wanted to be with Mr. Warren, to be who I was with him. When my dad was in his last illness, I had asked Mr. Warren to sign a book of poems to my dad. I still have it. It said, "To Elmer Milch, who is David's father, and I consider my good friend."

I couldn't get to my own feelings about my dad then. They were too big. But the specific ideas from the Jameses—that the totality of experience and behavior is all at play, that we must be hospitable to every story being available as material for rendering, that the good is what works, and that we can rewire ourselves by our behavior—would come to, and continue to, profoundly shape every aspect of how I lived. It would take me longer to get to writing about my dad, but I would do it eventually.

3.

Hustle

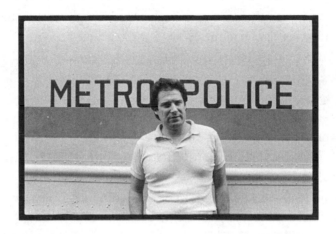

I GOT MY FIRST REAL JOB IN SCREENWRITING because there was a writers' strike in Hollywood. Jeff Lewis, my roommate at Yale when we were undergraduates, had gone to work for *Hill Street Blues*. He had been to law school and was a practicing lawyer for a bit first, so there was clearly some eagerness for people who were coming to this work by indirection. Jeff told his boss Steven Bochco about me and sent him some of my writing, and Steven invited me to come out to Los Angeles to write an episode. Steven had worked on *Columbo* and a few other shows but *Hill Street* was his first big success and it hadn't come easy. It was one of the first shows to tell stories over several episodes, serialized stories. The ratings the first season were terrible, but it set a record for Emmy nominations. After the second season his cocreator Michael Kozoll left the show, and then there was a strike. There was definitely a bit of luck at play that in that particular moment they couldn't ask any writer in the Writers Guild to write a script. The Writers Guild is the union that represents working screenwriters, but I wasn't in it yet, so they could ask me. Steven liked what I wrote and we liked each other, so when the strike got resolved he brought me on staff. I would never have had the career I had without Steven.

That first script I wrote was called "Trial by Fury," and going back to it now there is some satisfaction that on a basic level, as a piece of writing, it holds up. What is not strange, but let's say more relevant to our project here, is that the themes it explores, the dynamics it takes an interest in, are basically the stuff I'd keep going back to for the rest of my life. *Hill Street* had already existed for two seasons, became a hit in its second, and my episode would end up opening its third. The show famously started every episode with Sergeant Phil Esterhaus (the wonderful actor Michael Conrad) doing the roll call and going through the day's relevant items—here's a piece of the first roll call I ever wrote, the first dialogue of mine that ever aired on television:

ESTERHAUS

Item nine is a memo from Chief Daniels regarding
profanity in our dealings with the civilian populace—
which memo is also posted on the upstairs board.
People, I recognize downtown's tendency to be
unrealistic in these matters, but consider a complaint
I took yesterday from an elderly woman who had
been rendered assistance with her stalled vehicle by
one of our uniforms. Here was one of our own, going
the extra mile in the performance of his duty, yet he

was so accustomed to certain patterns of speech, that in arriving at the scene, he cheerfully inquired and I quote, "So what the bleep's wrong with your car, ma'am," said "bleep" allegedly causing complainant a severe episode of migraine.

Esterhaus turns to the blackboard. Earnestly pedagogical:

ESTERHAUS (cont'd)

Now I've assembled some terms you might try substituting for the swear words in question as you move through your daily routine. Now they won't come trippingly to your tongue at first, but with time and usage, you could find them becoming second nature. Your recourse to obscenity will then be fresh and vital when you encounter those situations and individuals for whom only obscenity will suffice. Now, the officer in question could have used the word "heck." Other more suitable terms: "drat," "shoot," "fudge," instead of the more common expletives usually associated with your street patois.

I didn't know in 1982 that I'd end up making shows known for profanity, but I did know I was interested in accounting for the divergence between what I considered a credible portrayal of the language of these characters and the way they had to talk because of the limitations imposed by network standards and practices. It's a show about cops and criminals and grown-ups, and how the networks required us to write the characters was not necessarily how they talked, but that can be okay if you figure out another way to honor the truth and vitality of the characters. And so that's what I was trying to do in that speech—to say the turns of language are going to feel different here, and there will be some artifice, but you'll get used to it and you might even come to like it. I wanted to draw attention to the artifice, and in turn to the energy of the language—you can make it "fresh and vital" by obscenity but also by making it a little silly. It's the same thing. To the extent that the thrust of my work has been toward ever more extreme varieties of language in their profanity or intricacy or strangeness, that has been to show, through the form of dialogue, the variety and ultimately the joy of the energy that's given to us all as humans to exchange and bear witness to.

There are two murders in the episode. A white nun and a Hispanic shopkeeper. The vast majority of the resources of the police department, and of the storytelling, go to the nun's storyline. The community is getting more and more agitated over the nun's rape and murder, but also the case isn't going great. They have guys in custody, but the nun dies in surgery and so the physical evidence is compromised. Another nun flubs the lineup. What the lead detective, Furillo, does to get one of the perpetrators to flip on the other is tell the prosecutor to release them, no holding, no bail, basically saying, "I'm gonna let this mob kill you if you don't confess." What you get out of that is the audience becoming complicit with Furillo, because the audience, like the mob, wants these guys punished, but they also want to feel smarter than the mob. You're rooting Furillo on—"Isn't that a clever solution?" And even when his girlfriend the defense attorney asks him, "Do the ends justify the means?," the audience is thinking, "Oh, *big time*."

Then two more things happen. The cops discuss the shopkeeper case and admit they're not gonna solve it. His wife and family aren't going to get justice. On some level the audience knows their neglect, and the neglect of the story itself plays a part in that. Then Furillo goes to confession. "Bless me, Father, for I have sinned." That's the end of the episode and the audience has to sit with it. The ends may justify the means but that doesn't mean it's not a sin. The law is provisional. It fails as often as it works. It's made up and improvised and inconsistent. I'd keep coming back to that too.

* * *

The C story in that episode isn't about a murder. Detective Belker brings in a male prostitute named Eddie Gregg who was based on my friend Eddie Grundy. Eddie Gregg was played by Charles Levin, a young curly-haired Jew, but the real Eddie was Black, and he would take the train from New York to New Haven to bring me my methadone. I didn't want my name on any lists so I had him get it for me. He turned tricks sometimes and he had dentures, and if he really liked somebody, he'd take the dentures out, "do 'em toothless." Once he was coming up to New Haven regularly he started spending time in the library and taught himself Latin and Greek so he could read the gay poets in the original. He'd just sit in Sterling laughing.

What I just did in the previous paragraph was juxtapose a series of details that in their extremity and seeming contradiction create what feels like a person. But also that's who Eddie was. The trick as a writer is how can you compress that layering of impressions so that the audience feels, "Oh, there's more than one thing going on with this guy." On one level, that's good writing because it's funny, or keeps the viewers' attention so they sit through the commercial and buy soap or whatever, but on another level, what the viewer is experiencing is, "Oh yeah, that's how people are."

With Eddie Gregg the character, he's all jokes—he introduces himself as Blanche DuBois, asks Belker to change the charge to "a tonier kind of bust." Then Belker gets a call from his mom and we only hear Belker's end of the conversation, but it becomes clear his dad is starting to lose his mind and how that's manifesting is he's acting like a dog (a symptom that, as far as I know, thus far I've been spared):

As Belker hangs up, obviously disturbed—

EDDIE

(has shown total involvement with the conversation)

How old is he?

BELKER

None of your business . . . He's eighty-two.

EDDIE

Senility's nothing to be ashamed of, you know.

BELKER

(flaring)

He's not senile!

EDDIE

It's part of life.

BELKER

(a growl)

Will you button it?

EDDIE

(unfazed)

My grandmother was senile, she had such fun on her birthdays. She'd open her present, then drift off, then look down, see her present and get happy all over again.

BELKER

(a portentous beat)

That's what my father does with his breakfast cereal.

A solemn and sympathetic chirp from Eddie.

What that storyline does in the midst of all these murders and failures is say, "You don't know where care is gonna come from." Same way you don't know where the danger might come. Of course reading it now, them talking about senility has another resonance. You don't know what things will come to mean.

* * *

When I came on to *Hill Street*, I had no background in entertainment at all. The James stuff was with the PBS station in Boston; this was an entirely different league. I was at the MTM building—the *St. Elsewhere* crew was on the first floor and *Hill Street* was on the second. I was in the writers' room with Steven, Jeff Lewis, Tony Yerkovich, Mark Frost, Karen Hall, and Michael Wagner and we'd tell stories and talk through ideas and figure out episodes. If there was a window washer going by, I felt I had to moon them. If Steven drove me home, there was also a good chance I was going to stick my bare ass out of the car. At least one time I pissed in someone's pencil cup. I made the other guys laugh.

I was gambling. A busy boy. I wasn't thinking about writing like this for my life. I was improvising. When I first went to work on *Hill Street*, not only would I carry around every cent that I made, but I'd carry it in silver dollars in an athletic bag. I'd fly to Las Vegas a lot of nights, gamble the silver dollars, then I'd walk around all day with the money. Nobody ever asked about the jingling.

But if you can write, you'll be okay. Steven put me on the accelerated course. He could tell that, within certain limitations, I was able to perform, to do certain things with elevated form. Once or twice that first season I had to ask him to front me my salary. He'd write me a check, and I would pay him back in cash. It was the cash, rather than the advance, that tipped him something was amiss. He asked me what was going on and I explained I was going to Vegas every night. He still lent me the money. I suppose he figured, "Let's just ride the horse," so that's what we did. Rita was still working back East. She was doing a documentary about an abortion clinic in Chester, Pennsylvania, that would air in the first season of *Frontline* on PBS and win an Emmy. She had no idea.

There's a prize called the Humanitas Prize that was started by a Paulist priest for scripts that are uplifting in their portrayal of the full human condition, and "Trial by Fury" won that prize. I took the check—a considerable amount of money, fifteen grand tax-free—and went out to the racing office at the racetrack and bought a horse. The fellow who was the moving spirit behind this prize was a polished priest, Father Ellwood Kieser. I have a certain ambivalence toward authority, and they gave me this prize and it seemed quite clear to me that Father Kieser had a rather secular bent. In my jaundiced view of the situation, Father Kieser was getting entrée for the polished fathers into show business. I more or less kept my mouth shut the first time, but then I won it again the next year. At this point I felt compelled to scandalize. I said, "I just want to tell Father Kieser that, having been a beneficiary of his munificence last year, I took that money and I bought a racehorse, which really is what I think Father Kieser would have probably wanted me to do. And I'm gonna use this money to buy another racehorse." I did everything but piss on the award. He was looking at me and smiling, his eyes set close together. And I was looking at him and I said, "Thank you very much, Father." A jerk.

Such immediate success seemed so inauthentic and accidental that there's an almost inevitable impulse to disown it, to invoke some ironic connection to it, because otherwise how do you account for the fact that you're a junkie? That you're a degenerate gambler? And whatever other forms of disreputable behavior you have? But in its way, that was considered a fulfillment of the horrible allegory of what happens to you when you move out to L.A.—the Bitch Goddess Success. "The filth of self, to be loved, must be clad in glory."

It wasn't a long exile before I started to generate enough recognition that it wasn't considered disreputable for me to be in L.A., but the mixture of messages that we all receive as children persists. A life in academia, even in letters, felt more respectable to my family. They looked down on L.A. On the other hand, the stuff I'd written was well received. And so it sort of suited all of us, I still got to be the fuckup. My brother was back in Buffalo, had married young to Linda, a Jewish girl also from Buffalo. They already had four great kids, he was already a surgeon like my dad, and I was the one who had left. In that way even the money and success became a part of my being a degenerate.

The transmutation of the idea of writing from being a hustle to being a sort of legitimate, organizing impulse did not occur in any immediate way and, surprisingly enough, the fact that I had taken those courses and spent that time working with Mr.

Warren was ultimately what legitimized the enterprise in my own imagination.

Mr. Warren had written a poem about Audubon, the naturalist and Frenchman who came to Kentucky and lived by himself in the woods for twenty years, painting birds. At first he'd kill them so he could get the details right. That section of the poem goes:

> He slew them, at surprising distances, with his gun.
> Over a body held in his hand, his head was bowed low,
> But not in grief.
>
> He put them where they are, and there we see them:
> In our imagination.
>
> What is love?
>
> One name for it is knowledge.

The mystical commitment that brought Audubon to live the way he lived, to feel that sense of awe when you enter into that state of being that you're testifying to the world's beauty and re-creating it somehow, was in part how Mr. Warren felt about writing. And that conception of the act allowed me to see the possibilities of screenwriting. My first and primary obligation as an artist was to the reality of the characters and their situation. And if I did nothing else or understood nothing else, as long as I did that right, I was going to do okay. I could trust myself to know how a character would behave in a particular situation, to "put them where they are," but I didn't know the lived facts of their past experience. I watch their behavior to infer what their past must have been to make them behave in the way they do now, and thus what the possibilities might be going forward. That commitment to knowing them, to getting them right, was love. Mr. Warren had given me the gift of understanding that this process—transforming something dark or painful into something joyful by seeing it and knowing it fully—is the proper function of art, whether it be poetry or prose or screenwriting.

It was that lesson, combined with meeting the people who would inspire the characters I write about, that revealed this form of storytelling as the organizing principle of my life.

The prostitute Eddie Gregg wound up being a recurring character on *Hill Street*, the first character that I created. I was with the show for five years, until it ended in 1987. I introduced a character named Norman Buntz, played by Dennis Franz, who was more explicit about the compromises he was willing to make as a cop. After Michael Conrad died, I had the new Sergeant Stan Jablonski close his roll calls with, "Let's do it to them before they do it to us," which to me felt truer to the enterprise.

One thing about a show with a big cast is that every actor gets a raise each year, which means that the show gets more expensive to make. By our fifth season, Arthur Price, who at that point ran MTM, the production company that made *Hill Street*, was very eager for Steven to cut costs by cutting a few characters from the show. Steven wouldn't do it. Steven's thinking was that the show was hitting the hundredth-episode mark anyway, which is the point at which a show starts to make real money from syndication, and we were going to make back our costs, and then some, for everyone involved. Arthur asked Jeff Lewis and me if we'd be willing to lose some characters and we said sure. Arthur fired Steven and made us executive producers. Steven was quite gracious about it in the press, probably at least in part because he'd still be making a good bit of money off the show as cocreator as long as we could keep it on the air, but he's also admitted the thing that hurt him was that Jeff and I didn't tell him when Arthur first approached us. He said he knew he would forgive me even then because he would never expect me to act with that kind of integrity, that it would be like being mad at someone for the color of their eyes. We cut five characters at the start of the sixth season, including the one played by Steven's wife. The show made it two more years.

* * *

Rita and I got married in 1982 in New York, and then I flew back to L.A. She moved for good in February of the next year and we had our first child, Elizabeth, in 1984. Rita had a long labor, and so while we waited I started making phone calls. Rita asked what I was doing and I said I was buying a horse. She looked at me and said, "Not enough action in the room, Dave?" in such a tone that even I knew to hang up the phone. I did end up buying that horse, though.

When Ben was born in 1986 we bought a house in Brentwood. There were six weeks when we were waiting to move that we lived in a hotel on Wilshire, and the tight quarters were wearing. I started drawing on the sheets, made up evil alter egos for the kids, named the evil kids Ruth and Isaac. We were lucky the Moreno Avenue house was ready when it was. It was this old Spanish house, built in the 1930s, and Rita made it beautiful. There were old palm trees all around and Rita planted what she tells me was a California pepper in the front, liquid amber trees in the backyard that changed color, a lot of vines and jasmine that grew up the walls. It was all alive. There was a guesthouse where she could paint and I could put people up, an old fountain with a sea monster–looking creature spitting out water that the kids played in, a swing set where I'd push them sometimes and sing, "He's got the whole world in his hands, he's got the whole wide world, in his hands." The success, or simply the money, created the circumstances in which we could proceed even though I was still using.

I would fly Eddie Grundy out to L.A. with his boyfriend Jesus. Another friend, Larry Mascetti, was my dealer at the Campus Dining Room in New York and after Columbia shut him down he'd come stay with us too. The kids loved him. They'd wake up and we'd go down to the kitchen and he'd already be cooking chicken and singing the old song "Sugartime" that my kids knew as the pizza bagel jingle but Larry would sing it about chicken, "Chicken in the morning, chicken in the evening, chicken at suppertime," and they didn't think that was at all strange.

I heard Richard Yates was sick by then and had no money (this was before wider audiences of people rightly rediscovered the greatness of his work) and I invited him out to L.A. to write TV treatments for me. I was giving him money, and he hated feeling beholden to anyone, but especially me. Any day we got together, I knew we'd have to spend at least one hour with him telling me I was wasting his talent and mine in a bullshit medium. There was some kind of payback going on, but also I wanted to take care of him. I put him and Larry together. Larry would drive Richard around and Richard would complain about Larry's cigars, but in their own way they became friends. The kids thought Richard's crotchety attitude was an act.

Kathleen Cleaver had been a student at Yale after her time leading the Black Panthers with Eldridge in Algeria and North Korea—we were actually the same age and she was one of the few people I knew for a fact had seen even more than I had, and she would come to stay with us. I had all of these wonderful people around me and I was working and had this young family and there was joy, but as an addict what I still found myself thinking was, "I'm fooling all of them." I was using money to distort my relationships with my old friends. I told myself most other writers in L.A. didn't really understand the world. I used the different parts of my life against each other, to tell myself I wasn't an authentic part of any of it, except for the work itself.

After *Hill Street* ended in 1987, career-wise I had what one might call a rough patch. I created a spin-off about Norman Buntz called *Beverly Hills Buntz* that was almost a comedy, with the character starting fresh as a private eye. His ambivalence toward the culture of L.A. mirrored some of my own, and people didn't seem to like that. Irony ultimately is not an adequate informing principle for long-term conduct. It can get you laid or it can get you through a short conversation, but that's about it. This was also in a period of network strategy where the show was made what's called "a designated hitter," meaning it aired in rotation with a few other shows. Sometimes a whole month would pass between episodes, which may have posed something of a challenge to viewership, also maybe people just didn't like it very much. But Hal Ashby directed the pilot and Ry Cooder did the music and Dennis Franz and the other actors did great work. They aired nine of the thirteen episodes we shot. In 1988 there was a TV movie called *Home Free* about a group home starring Michael Warren that was supposed to be a backdoor pilot, and that didn't get picked up either. We did another show called *Capital News* about a *Washington Post*–type paper that aired in 1990 with Lloyd Bridges, Mark Blum, and Wendell Pierce in one of his first big roles, so many great actors. We wrote thirteen episodes and they aired four of them.

When people have been bringing their efforts honorably and something fails, you feel like you've let them down. And given that whatever sense of feeling worthy of drawing breath I had was largely derived from my work, work not going well had cascading effects.

I'm wildly impatient and aggressive. Being an addict and using produced certain mutations and magnifications of those character traits that were already present within me.

We went to a party up in the Hills. I didn't want to go and, God help me, I used my own children as props. I said to their mother, "We'll bring the kids. We'll be there for twenty minutes and we'll pretend one of them is sick and we'll get out of there." We're the first ones there because we want to be the first ones out. I'm sitting there and talking to people, in utter misery on the sundeck, and I see this toddler in a walker heading right for the pool. I'm looking, and I remember saying, "Who's got that kid?" Boom, the kid goes into the pool upside down. I go off the deck, leap into the pool, get the kid.

Now I'm completely soaked. The host says, "Oh, that was so wonderful what you did. Let me take your clothes and put them in the dryer." Now I'm sitting there—fat and ugly and naked for an hour and I'm starting to get genuinely claustrophobic. I say to Rita, "As soon as these clothes are dry, we're out of here." Finally, the clothes come out, I get them on and I say, "Oh look at that, my kid's sick. Time to go." We go outside and it's stacked parking. There are like two hundred cars parked behind me. Now I'm the boss. I come back in and say, "Would it be possible for everyone to move their cars?" This one guy says, "I'll be happy to move mine. Mine's twenty-seven down if you get the others to move." I say to Rita, "Get the children and leave this to me." Rita knows: *I don't want to argue with him because he's got that look in his eyes, but something bad is about to happen.*

The kids get in the car. I drive down the cliff. Right down

the mountain. I did twenty-five-thousand dollars' worth of damage to the car. Went right between the trees and the kids are wide-eyed, bracing themselves—*It's kind of fun, I guess.* I say, "This is worth every cent." When you want to go, you go. As father Zorro said to little Zorro, you get in, you make your Z, and you get out.

There was another day Rita left me for about thirty minutes with Ben and Elizabeth and their two best friends, who were also brother and sister—two four-year-olds and two two-year-olds. They entertained themselves and I had money on the football game. Rita returned and pointed out that they had drawn all over the walls of the room we were sitting in and asked if I thought I would have noticed had they set themselves on fire.

*   *   *

In this same period, my friends started dying again. AIDS came and that wasn't great for intravenous drug users. The drugs themselves weren't great for your odds either. I had a writer friend named Mister Margulies in L.A. and one day his dad called and said he couldn't reach him. I was at work and asked Rita to go by his place to check on him, even though she was six months pregnant. She and the super go to the door and there is a smell and she knows. She calls me and says, "David, I can't go in there." So I drive over and go in and the first thing I see is that the television is on and there's this pair of legs watching the television. For a split second I think, "Everything's all right, he's just watching TV." Then I see that his head is the size of a rhinoceros and gray and I snap back to the smell. The stink in the room is unthinkable. He had gotten clean but then he picked something up and had to try it. I had to call his dad back with that. He says, "Can you find his prayer shawl and put it in his coffin?" I go back into the apartment and I'm burning coffee grounds for the stench and looking for his prayer shawl.

Michael Ruggere died. Larry Mascetti died. Eddie Grundy died.

I began to feel sick all the time, convinced I was dying. I was going to doctors for various tests—kidney disease, lupus, HIV. Every time, I'd make Rita get ready for bad news with me. If I wasn't at work I was in bed, stayed in my boxers. I was getting prescriptions from the doctors. Rita says what she remembers most was trying to keep the children quiet. A five-year-old, a three-year-old, and a newborn.

After the children were asleep we'd go out to the guesthouse where she painted and we'd talk, and sometimes I'd say, "Must we live in such a child-centered universe?" And Rita would say, "Well, yes, because we have three young children."

Then other times I'd say, "All I want is to be with you and the kids."

"We're right here. Come be with us."

But I felt I couldn't, or I wasn't, even when I was right there.

* * *

Then our boy got sick for real, my son Ben. His skin went pale and his lips were nearly blue. I noticed it first and I think for a minute Rita thought I was going Munchausen, starting in on the kids. But then she saw it too. We took him to the doctor and they said his red blood cell count was low, that it seemed like he had stopped producing them altogether. One potential cause for this was leukemia. Four adults had to hold him down for the spinal tap, his three-year-old body. There was no cancer, but they also didn't know what it was. He would have to get weekly blood transfusions until they could figure it out. I was type O, a universal donor. I gave my son my blood. I passed whatever screens they had then so they let me, and maybe I lied some. Rita's brother Gardy was Ben's match, he gave. Rita and Ben were going to the cancer ward at Cedars-Sinai every week. Surrounded by children who were very, very sick.

About three months in, he started making red blood cells again. They never figured out what it was, thought maybe it was a bad reaction to an antibiotic. The uncertainty of that made us more watchful with Ben, always wondering if it might come back.

Robert Penn Warren died in September of 1989, just after Ben got better. Ten years after my dad died. Earlier that year he had sent me a message that he wasn't well and asked me to come see him, and that was his last gift to me. I think he was trying to communicate to me that the way he had lived was sufficient, that the genuine experience of life's possibilities is coming unapologetically to the materials at hand.

To the extent that my relationship with Mr. Warren acted as a kind of balm on all sorts of pain, I can look back now and see that things got real raw real quick after that. I was so scared of what I might feel.

Putting this time into paragraphs, there's a sadness, it's exhausting; that feels true to what it was like, though the formal structure here gives it an organization that it lacked. You can look down the page and see that this section ends. We didn't know that at the time. My eldest, Elizabeth, had started kindergarten that year. She tells me all her memories from home then are gray. Olivia was an infant. The older two say the reason she's the upbeat one is because she doesn't remember.

In the summer of 1990, I went to rehab for the first time.

4.

Storytelling Is Not Therapy

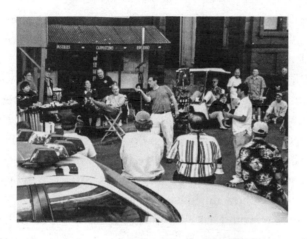

I DON'T REMEMBER A LOT FROM that trip to rehab, and I don't think I'd be spoiling too much to tell you the sobriety didn't stick. I do remember telling them, "I'm scared if I get sober, I'm going to hate my father." Aren't we all? I was either going to have to learn how to live with those feelings, or I wasn't. Even the willingness to admit that some things from my childhood were at play in my using, that was a forward development.

Absent action, all animals are sad. I had to get back to work.

One thing that was happening in the early 1990s was the networks realizing cable might be a bit of a threat. In particular, the fact that cable was showing movies that were more adult raised the question of whether the networks were losing ground by being so family-friendly. Or at least Steven Bochco was raising this question to various network executives because he saw an opportunity in it. He came to me and proposed working on another series together, pushing harder on some of the themes we had explored in *Hill Street*. That Steven was willing and even wanted to work with me again speaks to his kindness and generosity, and the kind of clear-eyed producer he was. He had a better sense of what I was capable of and what I needed than I did.

ABC bought what would become *NYPD Blue*. We found a rhythm together, where Steven could deal with the network, hiring, and casting, and I could focus on the stories and characters. Because we were trying to do something pretty different than what had come before, there was a lot of work to do with the network, a lot of negotiation about particular words and phrases, about how much of a butt cheek or a breast we could show. I likely would have committed a murder if I had been in those rooms at any length, but Steven could do it with patience while still pushing the ball forward.

At that time, television was typically seen as a reductive medium. Historically, the assumption had been that because the experience of television was in the home, presumably where people are more distracted, an audience is not willing to invest emotionally in ways that test the extent of its commitment to the materials, or its willingness to experience unpleasant or conflicting emotions. We wanted to challenge that assumption. But when the show's about to come out, if Steven Bochco gives an interview and says television has been assumed to be a medium that people don't want to make any emotional investment in and we're going to challenge that assumption, nobody's going to give a shit. If he says we're doing nudity and dirty words the likes of which network TV has never experienced, he's on the front page. That's why Steven had a plane. He understood how to frame the issue to make our intentions accessible.

I had written two scripts already, but all that negotiation gave me what would end up being an extra year or so to do research. At the start of that, not knowing how much time I would actually have, I talked to two reporters in New York, Jimmy Breslin and Michael Daly, and asked them who the best detective in the city was. They both named the same guy. A homicide detective named Bill Clark who worked out of Queens but was sent all around the city because he was so good in the interrogation room. He had helped get the David Berkowitz confession in the Son of Sam case.

So I asked Bill if I could spend some time with him. As soon as we met, I knew this show was about to get a whole lot better.

In a certain way, what you're doing in evaluating somebody you meet is drawing on your own past experience of other people and getting a sense of what good faith they're able to bring to the exchange. Bill was watching me too. Early on, I could see him deciding how much to tell me. There's a process that happens if you open your imagination to the particular truths of a different person and a different environment, to try to give your imagination to what you don't know. It's humbling but also enormously rewarding. One way or another you're saying, "Teach me"—you have to be willing to learn.

It was coming to know Bill that made it possible for me to develop a much different sort of specific lived understanding of what it meant to be a cop. Bill took it personally. He loved his block. When I was first riding with him and he would see graffiti, I would see him start to get aggravated. He'd say, "You can't let that happen, this is where we live. You let people do that, then they're going to feel they can do something else." If he saw somebody dumping garbage, he stopped. He'd get the guy and say, "Pick the garbage up," because this was his house. I'm not saying whether I think that was right or not, whether it might have other social or political consequences. I was observing the behavior. People who are good at what they do have their own self-respect. If you communicate your respect for them, then they give up their secrets. Then they're able to acknowledge their secret pride.

Bill had an earnest and honorable intention allied with a willingness to undertake whatever effort would bring about the intended purpose; a willingness to shed the limits of what might be considered correct behavior in order to accomplish what he felt to be a final good. There are situations and behaviors that are grounded in motives beyond the law. The failure to accept that fact is a disservice to humane results. One of the things I found most edifying about Bill was his willingness to accept that truth, to honor it, and not to exclude it as shaping the way he moved in the world.

One of the first cases Bill and I talked about was one that Bill had worked where a kid was sexually violated and later murdered. An eighteen-year-old had killed an eight-year-old, and Bill's task was to make the perpetrator feel that Bill understood. He said, "Look, you didn't want to. God knows you didn't want to kill him. You had sex with him. Now you're afraid his parents . . . he's going to tell somebody. You did what you had to do." Bill's job as a detective was, through language, to bring the act, as much as possible, within the pale of acceptable human behavior, so that this kid would confess.

You do what you have to do. The good is what works. The thing that interested me most about interrogations, that I knew would be fruitful for dramatization, is that everyone is lying, cop and suspect both, and everyone knows they're lying. Then, through the lies, through the act of lying, sometimes you get to a version of the truth, which was previously shaped by, and afterward will once again move through, all sorts of additional systemic distortions.

I've seen more than one murderer confess and ask if Bill could stay in the room when their lawyer got there. Bill's gift was making them feel like he was the only person who really understood them, or the only person who was telling them the truth. Bill would say he only went hard to get a confession when he knew someone was guilty. I've also seen Bill go after cops he thought put the wrong guy behind bars, leaving weekly messages reminding them that the wrong guy was eating prison food.

The way that the series developed, Bill and I would work together conceiving the stories, then I would work on the drafts and Bill would give me notes. I would fly out to New York to spend time with him. He'd introduce me to other detectives, they'd all tell me stories. I gained about fifty pounds in this period of research because we were taking guys to steak joints for every meal and I knew it would rub them the wrong way if I didn't eat. When Bill would come to L.A. he would stay at our house. We'd watch *Jeopardy!* every night with my kids and compete against each other. Bill and I became real friends, best friends, and in all sorts of ways it changed both of our lives.

With Bill, my city miles helped us understand each other—he knew I wasn't an innocent. But we were also still working, and we both got to bring it all to the table. Bill had such doubleness too. For all the bodies he'd seen, the things he'd done, he was also the sweetest person I had ever met, with animals, with children. He had been in Vietnam and seen burned bodies and been shot at, but when he'd well up was when he talked about his patrol dog, Mox. He had hundreds of birds. He loved antiques. I was more integrated with Bill than anyone since Judgy. Everything was in play.

My kids were still young then; our eldest was only eight when Bill first came to stay, and with him being in our house, I got to be engaged in front of them in a different way. We all liked it. At first Bill would try not to talk about murders around them, but I'd tell him to go ahead. So that was us around the kitchen table. He taught Ben and Olivia how to ride bikes. He and Rita became very close—it was the first time Rita had another adult to talk to about the full Dave experience.

That full experience, which was never simple, got more complicated in those first years of *NYPD Blue*. The money meant I could buy more horses, which I did. One of them was Gilded Time, who would become the best two-year-old in the country for a bit. He was racing in the Breeders' Cup in Florida and so I flew about sixty people down there for a race. My business manager calls and says, "Not for nothing, if the horse loses, those people are stranded because you don't have the money to fly them all back." So then I call my agent and say, "Get me a script to fix because this fucking horse is no cinch." I'm in my hotel room doing rewrites on *Bad Boys*, because it was originally intended for I think Jon Lovitz and Dana Carvey and now they wanted me to revise it so that it made sense for Will Smith and Martin Lawrence. The producer Don Simpson is berating me over the phone like, "What'd you say you wrote for? *The Munsters*? I don't give a shit. I owe it to a film to have at least six writers work on it." Then the horse wins. We get back to L.A., and they ask me to do some more work on the script.

"I'm good."

"What if we tell Don to tone it down?"

"Tell him to go fuck himself. Tell him to get hit by a fucking bus. My horse won. I'm out."

I was working all the time. I worked seven days a week. If I wasn't at work, I was at the racetrack. What you find is that you're working at such an accelerated pace, you relax the same way. You've got to bet ten thousand or twenty thousand dollars a race. Or if you start betting ten thousand dollars, at the end of the day you're betting forty thousand. I bet so much money that if I put it into the machines where the odds are figured, it'd distort the price. It'd ruin my own odds. What personal book-makers do is book the bet themselves. They lay it off with organizations elsewhere, and those organizations book the bets themselves. Pari-mutuel just means "among ourselves." It's French. Betting amongst ourselves. The name I used with the bookies was David Mary. I'd have to say my name with each bet so they could track it. "David Mary, Santa Anita sixth race, exacta box, the two horse and the three horse." David Mary, bet, David Mary. I'd bet on football, basketball. Weekends could really go one way or another depending on how I did. So could weekdays. I did a million dollars in a day, more than once. How many times depends on who I'm lying to. Bill and Rita would exchange a look when we got home for the day: *What kind of mood's he in?* If things were up, we had fun. If things were down, they'd all eat dinner as quickly and silently as they could and then go hide.

* * *

When we were casting the show, we knew we wanted Dennis Franz to play Sipowicz, but he was somewhat reluctant given it would have been the twenty-seventh cop on his résumé. At first he said no. I told him don't worry, Sipowicz is getting shot in the first episode, just do the pilot with us. I knew from the jump

Sipowicz was gonna live, but I wanted Dennis to start playing him before I told him. He really believed he didn't want to spend years of his life playing another cop. I had a feeling once he got to know Sipowicz he wouldn't mind sticking around.

Casting the other lead, John Kelly, was trickier. Steven initially wanted Jimmy Smits for the part, but he was shooting a movie in Morocco. There was a guy who had played an Irish gang leader on *Hill Street*, David Caruso, who kept coming up. I wasn't necessarily on board. David's method was to draw the camera into himself. It's very, very effective, because it causes the audience to begin to imagine what the character's process is. But I worried the audience would be so engaged in that process with Kelly that it would bleach the rest of the world of its reality. As usual I turned out to be wrong. No one could have done that part as well as David did.

As we got closer to the premiere date, some religious organizations and "parent" groups really started going after the show. The depth of feeling from the opposition, particularly among the fundamentalists, was a surprise to me. I remember they put us on *The Phil Donahue Show*, and the vituperation was unexpected. We received more than a few death threats. Strangely, if enough people accuse you of having serious intentions, after a while you start to feel like a serious person. I had come to really love the show by then. The work felt important. The breakthrough in terms of language was really a substantive contribution. It made the show more believable, and it helped me with the rhythms of my writing. The recourse to obscenity was fresh and vital—this world's own true language was revealing itself.

Steven was prepared to go to bat. One of his greatest gifts was to know when to pick a fight, to know which fight could lead to a much larger victory. The fights that he picked, over language, over nudity, made the show better, and they made enormous ratings. I think if you sat him down and he had to tell the truth, some of those fights were orchestrated at least in part to gain some kind of attention. The show finally aired, and it was a hit, top show in its time slot, top three shows of the week, even with a third of ABC affiliates initially refusing to air it. Critics saw and appreciated what we were doing with the medium and the stories we were telling.

Tuesday at ten P.M. became a very important time in our house. I expected everyone to be watching the show. There was one night someone called at about 9:56, and Rita picks up in case it's something important. I snap, "Who the fuck is that?" I throw the remote across the room. She gets off before the opening credits end. It was my mom I think. All three of our kids were still under ten years old when the show started, but when the night's episode was over I'd go to each of their rooms and ask them what they thought. "It was good, Dad. Good episode."

Even with the success, and in part because of it, we were having problems on set. David Caruso, along with every other actor on the show, was doing remarkable work, but his process for getting to his character often involved questioning the writing. "Who wrote this shit? I'm not gonna say it." I would have to justify the dialogue to him. It didn't feel like we were exploring the scene together, with each other or the other actors; it felt like I was going to set to convince him to say his lines. Kelly too was an isolate, a withdrawn guy, and I genuinely believe this was David's way of getting to him, and the results were very compelling work. Sometimes he'd leave the set and isolate in his trailer. I suspect, like many of us, he was trying to duplicate certain aspects of the environment of his youth. But it was tough, it short-circuited what I felt should be a more shared experience. I got the sense that David primarily saw our show as a stepping-stone to a film career, and I took offense to that. He developed a not inaccurate belief that I was writing more for Dennis Franz. I felt that David didn't necessarily stay in the scene for his colleagues' close-ups. That too offended me, and I let him know. We were both looking for something in the other that we weren't getting, maybe a kind of gratitude, but we kept not getting it, and getting pissed off instead.

One day, during one of these arguments on the set, I started to feel an odd pressure in my chest. The guy's telling me the scene is shit, or that's what I'm hearing, and I'm thinking, "I am *not* going to give him the satisfaction of dropping dead in front of him. I am not going to give it up." I manage to extricate myself and walk over to Bill and say, "Take me to the fucking hospital." Turned out I was having a heart attack.

What they ultimately found was that one of my arteries was ninety-seven percent blocked, another one ninety, but at least there was one okay one that was only seventy percent. So I told Rita, and we told the kids, and I went in for surgery. Rita has ten thousand varieties of silence. She was very present to the degree I would let her be, but I wouldn't let her stay the night. I told her to go home to the kids. I was gone at work most of the time, so my being out of the house wasn't news. If Rita was away, that's what would have been scary, that meant something was wrong, and I couldn't bear it. They visited once when I was in the hospital, and I think that was enough for all of us. I didn't like them to see me like that, tubes in my arms and nose. They were little kids.

I was forty-seven then, and my body and my doctors were telling me some things were going to have to change. All I could think was, "Don't make me stop working." I started exercising every day, and totally changed my diet, and eventually I lost about fifty pounds. Steven and Bill and all of our other producers let me keep going, helped make it possible so I could. Bill, especially, started thinking as much as a TV writer as a cop when he would tell me his stories: "Here's something I think we could use."

Between our first and second seasons, in what was supposed to be some quieter recovery time, David asked for more money and time off to do movies. Then, in the midst of those negotiations, he decided he would like to leave the show no matter what. At that juncture, everyone involved agreed that would probably be for the best. So while I was recovering from an additional heart surgery, because another artery had collapsed, I had to revise the first six scripts of our second season and figure out how to write John Kelly out and bring a new lead detective into the show.

When the news broke that David was leaving, it became a big story. We were the biggest drama on television, and David was the breakout star, and now he seemed to be walking away. The audience felt betrayed, and they needed a target for their resentment. This was directed in part at Steven, the network, and me for failing to find a solution, but people really went after David—he was perceived as greedy, disloyal. What people were actually doing was grieving their relationship with the character John Kelly. They were pissed off that someone they had grown to like was leaving their life, and David became the target for all those feelings. Those feelings have sometimes complicated the audience's experience of David's work since, but he still does great work.

Before I go forward, one more story about David Caruso. Ten years later, when my eldest was heading to Yale and looking at the Southern California admit list ahead of some event, she sees the name of David Caruso's daughter, they were the same year. She says to me, "Is this going to mess me up? Is she going to hate me?" I say, "It's a big school. Don't worry about it."

The first week of school, they meet at a party, and they become best friends. Six weeks in, my daughter gets up the courage to tell me on the phone. All I can say is, "No kidding." That summer, Greta stayed with us on Martha's Vineyard. She's amazing, funny, tough-minded. And she and my daughter have this ease with each other, and you realize part of where it comes from is they have this shared understanding that their fathers have been tough to love and they love them anyway, and no one else can know that about them the way they know it about each other. They lived in an apartment together their junior and senior years of college. David and I would see each other again for the first time at their graduation. He was on *CSI: Miami* then, so he was doing pretty well for himself. We smiled, shook hands, and he said to me, "You know I saw you recently on the freeway."

"Oh you did?"

"The first thing I notice, this guy still has a nicer car than I do."

"This is something, isn't it?"

"This is something."

Our daughters have known each other for twenty years. They're still best friends. It's a gift. When I think about David now, that's what I think about.

* * *

In the second season, Jimmy Smits joined the show as Detective Bobby Simone. Having a hit is so rare, and at the time, no one knew if the change would doom us, if that would be the end. But the show went on, and it stayed successful, and I would say the work got even better as the histories of the characters themselves accumulated.

That second-season New York shoot, that was a fun time. We knew by then things were going to work out. Dennis and Jimmy were getting along great. The *New York Post* did an article about Bill and Jimmy riding along with cops, so Bill was happy. We'd stay at the Regency Hotel and I was giving out a lot of money. If I walked by you in the hall, the odds were pretty good you'd get a hundred dollars out of it. This made people quite kind. I went out and bought some loafers at Prada. I didn't usually care about that sort of thing but these were very comfortable. I was with Rita and I said, "Let's get a pair for everybody. Call the wardrobe department and get everyone's shoe size."

Bill and I could get into trouble together though. If someone cut us off in traffic, we'd go about twenty miles out of our way to make them see the error of their ways. I once ripped off someone's windshield wiper. The problem with that is then you end up giving them five thousand dollars cash to avoid a lawsuit. Rita would try to warn me, saying, "One day someone is going to shoot you." So I wrote an episode where a guy got into a road rage beef and his wife got killed instead. Rita took that as my rejoinder, but I hope what I was trying to say was that would have been my deeper fear.

The heart problems didn't go away. I'd had angioplasties, but then I had to have a stent. Then I'd have more pain and have to have another angiogram. The camera goes up through your leg and travels through your veins all the way to your heart, like you're Martin Short in that old movie (that happens to be a good movie). While I was having those heart operations, I was pretty down about it, in particular the idea that I might die. It seemed so cruel, and therefore to me so much more likely, that when things were really starting to go well, they might be taken away. I told Rita, "I want them to do everything they can to keep me alive, and if this really goes south, I want you to give me the biggest possible funeral." The doctors suggested I see a psychiatrist who specialized in middle-aged patients depressed about having heart disease, to be distinguished I suppose from the elderly people who are cheerfully skipping around having received the news.

But that's how it happened that when I was working on *NYPD Blue* it was also the first time I was in any kind of ongoing therapy. In the course of that therapy, I was diagnosed with bipolar disorder and put on medication, and I mean I was put on a lot of medication. Initially Depakote and trazodone. They tried Lamictal but I got the telltale rash that you can get which means you should not take Lamictal. They added Zoloft to the mix. For a long time I was reluctant to go on lithium because I was worried it would impact my writing, but eventually lithium joined the party too. My doctor still tells me he thinks I might be one of the most undermedicated people he's ever treated.

So for the first time in my life I was getting some treatment for things that had been going on. The bipolar disorder gave a name to so much of how I'd been. The times I'd insist the kids and I go buy a hundred Egg McMuffins and hand them out door-to-door to the neighbors, then my offense at the subsequent horror and confusion on our neighbors' faces as I put unasked-for Egg McMuffins in their hands. For Rita especially, things made a lot more sense. The doctors confirmed what she had felt for a while now—I was nuts. But they also agreed with her on another crucial point, one I had long resisted—there were other ways I could live.

During *NYPD Blue*, the ways I could engage with my own life and my past were evolving, and as the series went on, that started to happen more and more through my work on the show itself. As a writer, you're only halfway conscious of a lot of that stuff as you're writing, if that much, and that's as it's supposed to be. I was doing the work. I knew that work was good for me. But things find their way in, and you have to be open to it. The satisfaction of doing good work is inseparable for me from the things it makes you brave enough to do.

Mark Twain used to say that any character he wrote he was meeting for the second time, because he met them first on the river. That's how his time working on a riverboat shaped him, why he took his name from it. The character Sipowicz was based in large part on Bill and his work as a detective. Sipowicz was also inspired in part by my dad. Sipowicz doesn't do well with uncertainty or the unfamiliar. He had to exist in a very narrow and familiar sort of band of experience, and my understanding of him in that way was largely based on my experience with my dad.

One night my dad came home and a grateful patient had given him a record player. He went into the study and he looked at the record player in there like it was a crouching beast. Because he was an alcoholic and you couldn't disrupt his fucking routine. This was something new in the place where he had his drink before dinner. He just looked at this thing and said, "What the fuck is that?"

I said, "It's a record player, Dad. Frank Sinatra, you know."

He said, "I don't know anything about any goddamn record player."

Boom, through the window.

And that's Sipowicz too. When I met Sipowicz I was in some sense meeting him for a third time, through my meetings with him by way of my father and Bill. There's also a kind of rhetorical excess that is endearing and tends to defang the character. Sipowicz is very self-enclosed and in many ways a frightening character, but what purges the character a little bit of what is frightening about him is his idiosyncratic use of language and these islands of gentleness we see in him.

Another way I came to know Sipowicz was through the actor who played him, Dennis Franz. What Dennis was very good at was leaving room for the audience to understand more about Sipowicz than he understood about himself. Working with an actor on a set is like being in a confessional: What're they able to hear? What can I tell them, or what do they know they can tell me? You have to have a sense of what the soul with whom you're in communication is able to hear. You need, as well, a proper humility about what you are able, responsibly, to communicate. And that transaction, if it's honorably undertaken, is very delicate and humbling. You try to distill and extract what's central and useful in what you're conveying. It seems to me that it's the final distillation, the final communication and discovery of your intention—a last purifying of intention. It's sometimes useful to think of the exchange as a joining in prayer. The effort to understand the character's essence. You feel as if you're sending the person on a journey and hoping that you've done your part in preparing them. Dennis and I got to pray together a lot, for a long time, and it was a deep blessing.

Sipowicz's journey as a father carries throughout the series. The very first season, Andy Jr., played wonderfully by Michael DeLuise (who had his own experiences with a father who loomed large), shows up to tell his dad he's getting married even though he's only eighteen and hasn't seen his father in five years. Sipowicz tracks down this woman, figures out she's a scammer, and uses the seven hundred dollars Andy Jr. had wanted to borrow to get her a ring to pay this woman off to leave him. He's protecting his son and causing him pain and loving him and being a jerk all at once.

Sipowicz got sober before I did. His going on and off the wagon, and his trying to figure out how to be a father and how to properly integrate his past and his present, that's some of the work I'm proudest of. I feel some hesitation drawing these connections with my own life because ultimately the world of the work is separate—it's not me. Sipowicz is his own creation, the world of the show is its own organism, but it's all material for rendering. The more I opened myself to that, the better I could be.

In the third season, Sipowicz shows his son how to take a corner, and in a certain way it is the high point for Sipowicz, his training Andy Jr. to be a cop. It's just at this time that Sipowicz's second son, Theo, is born. It is the moment that he's able to embrace the idea that the past is recoverable and relivable, and that it's possible to make better everything he failed to do as a father in all those years when he was alienated from his first son. He now feels as if he's going to get a chance to make up for it in teaching Andy Jr. how to be a cop and, by extension, how to live, and then get to do it all with Theo. Then Andy Jr. gets killed, and it nearly breaks Sipowicz. He goes off the wagon, his wife has to kick him out. But Sylvia is still there, his second son is still there, his partner, Simone, is still there, and by being there they are asking him to live.

In our fourth season, in an episode called "Taillight's Last Gleaming," Sipowicz has a series of dreams wherein his dead son comes back to life. I wrote those dreams after I had a dream about my dad in which the situation was reversed. He was alive. Rather than Sipowicz coming to a dead son, I came to my dead father. It was nearly twenty years since he had died. I was in a restaurant, and I saw him sitting in the restaurant, and I said, "Dad, that's, how—you know, it's good to see you, how are you? Dad, you know, it's great, it's great to see you."

"I'm doing pretty good, I'm doing pretty—I'm dead, I'm dead, you know, but I feel pretty good."

"Geez, I'm so glad, because I always, whatever the reason, I had never been doing that great, you know, when you were alive. I'm so glad to be able to see you again, to let you know things are well. I'm married. I have children."

"What's that supposed to mean?"

"It doesn't mean anything. I'm just glad to tell you, let you know this."

"So am I supposed to feel guilty, that you didn't, you couldn't do well when I was alive?"

"No. I'm just saying."

"What? Are you going to break my balls? I'm dead. I'm dead. I got my own problems."

"Never mind. Good to see you."

"Yeah, go fuck yourself."

So I woke up and I didn't know what to make of that. Within five minutes the same bullshit that used to go on between us when he was alive was going on in the dream, and I was so sad.

In the show, the first dream comes right after the credits, and you see Sipowicz walking into this crowded diner, so for the first few beats the audience doesn't know it's a dream. Sipowicz sits down at the counter next to this trucker, but then in the seat beyond he sees his dead son:

SIPOWICZ

Could I switch seats with you?
It'd be a big favor.

TRUCKER

Yeah.

SIPOWICZ

Appreciate it.

(to Andy Jr.)

Son?

ANDY JR.

Hey, Pop.

SIPOWICZ

Aw, Andy. Can I give you a kiss?

ANDY JR.

Will they throw us out?

SIPOWICZ

Oh my God.

(hugging)

I can't believe it's you.

ANDY JR.

How you been? How's Theo?

SIPOWICZ

Oh, God, he's—he's wonderful. He had some health questions, but he—he's fine.

ANDY JR.

And Sylvia's good?

SIPOWICZ

She's wonderful. She's a wonderful mother. You know,
I'm trying to understand what's going on.

ANDY JR.

You know, I'm—I'm dead, but I'm—I'm doing all
right.

SIPOWICZ

I, uh—I wish we'd have seen you sooner. We had a lot
of sorrow with your death.

ANDY JR.

Pop, we didn't see each other too much when I was
alive.

SIPOWICZ

What's your inference with that?

ANDY JR.

No, I'm just saying?

SIPOWICZ

Nobody says I didn't make any mistakes.

ANDY JR.

I would've liked to have seen the baby and Sylvia too.
That's all I'm saying.

SIPOWICZ

I took you for breaking balls, my not seeing you
growing up.

ANDY JR.

It's a little late about that, Pop.

SIPOWICZ

I wish to hell they'd let you come over there, Andy.
The little guy, huh, well, he's a real pisser. And in
forty ways he reminds me of you. I never say that to
Sylvia 'cause of the upset. Did I just ruin something
now with my nature?

ANDY JR.

No. Anyways, um, I gotta go.

SIPOWICZ

If I offended anybody, let 'em know I try to curb it.

ANDY JR.

Yeah, I—I don't know how it works. I love you, Pop.

SIPOWICZ

Any opportunity, any modification on my part—

ANDY JR.

Love to Sylvia and the baby.

SIPOWICZ

Take good care of yourself as you can.

(*To the trucker who had been between them*)

My son.

TRUCKER

He's a good-looking boy.

> SIPOWICZ

I did something here. They pulled him.

> TRUCKER

Is that it for him, or is he coming back?

> SIPOWICZ

I can't talk no more.

> TRUCKER

Should've talked across me.

> SIPOWICZ

I can't talk no more. I'm finished.

Sipowicz is the audience's surrogate in the scene, trying to figure out what's going on. The trucker is this third seemingly benign presence, first obliging Sipowicz, noticing how good Andy Jr. looks, asking if he'll come back. "Should've talked across me," that's the line that leaves open the chance there's something else going on, though I didn't know what it was. You can use surrogates that way too. You give the audience a place to identify, then you introduce another variable and it leaves a way to open the whole thing up.

At the end of the episode, there's a second dream, now in a bar. One temptation as a storyteller might be to give the audience the satisfaction of Sipowicz learning from the first dream and changing, being different with his son this second time, not getting caught up in the same stuff. And Sipowicz wants so badly for his old son and his new son to meet.

I found in writing it that I couldn't satisfy that wish, for Sipowicz or for the audience. In the second dream he still can't let go of that fixation, that Andy Jr. be with Sylvia and Theo, and so he and Andy Jr. get into it again. Andy Jr. says, "Think seeing me murdered is gonna make a happy memory?" Sipowicz realizes that's where they are, the bar where Andy Jr. was murdered, and then his son's dead again in front of him. Then the trucker from the first dream is there, and Sipowicz starts in on him, "We're gonna be lifetime companions?" You hear Andy Jr. say, "That's Jesus Christ, Dad. Congratulations pissin' off Jesus Christ." The trucker takes Andy Jr.'s body on his shoulder, carries him, and says to Sipowicz, "What did I tell ya? Talk through me. Talk through me."

When I write, I go back and I read everything again the next morning, to say, "Does that feel right?" Does that feel right? Does it feel like he would've said that, even if I don't know why he said it? When I had that dream and tried to write out of the feelings that came from my dream, I didn't know what the dream meant. Then, in writing the first dream, I didn't know who the trucker was, other than he was a trucker who was between Sipowicz and his son, which was good for the scene with the audience. If your emotional commitment to the materials is genuine, you trust that somehow a meaning will come to all the characters. You simply try and get the people right, because if you get the people right, everyone is connected. I felt that that truck driver had a right to be in the bar because he'd been in the diner, and I had no sense of him other than that. These are elements of Sipowicz's consciousness talking to themselves, and it's he who chooses to assign the identity of Christ to this random figure from the first part of his dream. It wasn't until Sipowicz's son said "that's Jesus Christ" that I knew that's who it was. The actor who plays the trucker is Jim Beaver. He would later play the character Ellsworth on *Deadwood*. The "talk through me" becomes like a call for acceptance—accept the space between, that your first son is gone, that you must keep going now with your new baby without him. That's your chance for happiness now, it's not going to come by wishing you got to have them together.

In the process of writing that story, I came to a much fuller kind of emotional appreciation of what had gone on in the dream with my dad. It was simply a way of being with him again, a way of being present with him. In psychology, those are called completion dreams and they are a kind of forgiveness. My dad never met my kids. I've never been with my dad and my children. He never saw a single thing I've written on television. It doesn't do me any good to wish it were otherwise. Even though the content of the dream seems to express a continuing alienation, in fact what you're doing is recalling in forgiveness the way things were and not letting it destroy you, just remembering it the way it was. Writing that storyline for Sipowicz allowed me to appreciate that. That's what art lets you do.

* * *

Now those are only two scenes in that episode. In the very first scene, even before the credits, Lieutenant Fancy and his wife get pulled over in Staten Island by two white uniform cops for a busted taillight and the cops pull guns on him. Even after he says he's on the job, they're holding their guns on him and his wife. For the rest of the episode, you're following Fancy dealing with that experience. The next day, Fancy has the cops come to his office at the station, and the uniform cop Szymanski won't apologize. He says, "I can't help what you think. Till I have control of a situation out there, how'm I supposed to know what I'm dealing with?" So Fancy decides he's gonna call in a favor to have the cop transferred to Bed-Stuy. A writer named David Mills wrote that episode, he was a producer on the show by then. That plotline came out of David coming to me and saying, "I want to do a story where Fancy gets off on being mean-spirited. I'm sick of Black people only being portrayed either as criminals or as saints." I said okay, go write it.

I got to know David Mills around the start of the second season, the fall of 1994. The Humanitas Foundation had invited me to give a talk to a group of aspiring writers in November of that year—"Human Values in Entertainment Writing: The Challenges and the Pitfalls." I talked about writing a racist character like Sipowicz and being able to acknowledge that I enjoy writing that part of his character. In the course of that I talked about why I thought it might be more difficult for Black writers to succeed in network television. I said that because a Black person has experienced a sense of otherness in relation to the dominant society, which is traumatic, I thought it could be a complicated process for a Black writer to come to the kind of emotional equanimity that is necessary to write a whole bunch of characters for a show in which the majority of the characters are white, which was most network television shows at that time, and that to the extent that he does that, he may feel that he's writing away from or betraying his own experience. I was describing what I felt was a difficult emotional process, a more complicated process. I said if I'm honest with myself it's also the case that a Black writer probably has to be ten percent better than a white writer for me to hire them because I'm thinking to myself, "Every fucking time we're going to talk about a story I'm going to get into a Black and white thing, and it's going to take me too much time, and I'm going to have to worry about his or her feelings." Those are all unconscious feelings that operate in me, and it would be absurd not to acknowledge that that happens. Now, just one problem with that is my insisting in the next breath that I believe in a meritocracy—

that's a bit hard to square with saying a Black writer has to be better to make me willing to deal with my own discomfort.

The Washington Post got a recording of the talk and published an article. I had to speak with the network PR people, the president of the network had a talk with Jesse Jackson, it was a big thing.

After the talk and the article, David Mills, who I didn't know then, wrote me a letter. He said, "Congratulations on guaranteeing the future employment of so many mediocre white motherfuckers." What David pointed out in this letter was that even if he took me at my word that I was just talking about different writers' emotional processes, I had to know people were going to use my saying that as their own excuse for not hiring people. That they would say, "Even Milch admits he doesn't want to deal with that bullshit." Also, Mills said in his letter, I wasn't doing a full service to my characters if they were only drawing from the well of one kind of experience for their stories. I figured, well, I've got to meet this Mills guy. It turned out he had previously submitted a script that another producer had read and passed on. I found it, and it was good. I wound up hiring him.

Another conversation that came out of that talk was with James McDaniel, who played Lieutenant Arthur Fancy. He asked me to consider whether I had stopped short of giving his character the full expression of humanity that I gave to Sipowicz or others, in part because it was a more complicated process for me to gain access to his character's experience. And it was, and if I didn't admit that and push harder to do it, I wasn't meeting my full obligation as an artist or as James's collaborator. It is a complicated process, but it's a problem of spirit that can become a problem of technique. I was getting the chance to make that effort every week, and so maybe the real difference is not that it's more or less complicated for any kind of writer to write someone different from them but who's getting the chance to try. I said to James, "We might be in some trouble right now, but ultimately some good may come out of it." I look back at the stories we told after that, and James McDaniel's work, and there isn't much else like it. Our show was structured in such a way that the two main guys were always going to be the focus, but James McDaniel could do anything.

So David Mills and I were working on that episode and this Fancy storyline together—he'd been on the show three seasons by then, this was his ninth script. The way we did the show, Bill and I would talk through the story with the writer who was assigned, they'd do a draft, and then Bill and I would give notes and the writer and I would revise it together. Then once we were shooting I'd make more revisions, working with the actors on set to change lines or realizing we needed to add or take something away, and then in the editing room I'd do some final things, cutting lines or changing the order of scenes or losing one or two altogether. All of that's part of letting the episode exist as an organic living thing. In the early draft of that story, after Fancy has this cop transferred to Bed-Stuy, the cop comes to him and says basically, "Oh, because you took my stopping you as a race thing, now you're gonna ruin my life." And Fancy says, "Well, it's like you said, you pull somebody over out there, it's no telling who you're dealing with."

As we worked on the story, it seemed to me that that was too easy, that if we left it there with Fancy, we weren't being true to his character. I felt that given another chance, the character of Fancy as we knew him would be larger-spirited than that, because he is a character who is very hard on himself, who holds himself to a very high standard even at the expense of his own pleasure. David felt, fuck that, it's more important culturally to tell this story and leave Fancy being a bad guy to send a message that this was a mainstream show that was not going to be afraid to show a Black guy in a negative light. I said this was not a show whose intentions were cultural—this was a show whose intentions were creative and I wasn't going to betray my sense of the character's complexity to execute a sociological intention. We went around and around and around about that, and I won because I was the boss.

I said go and write another scene with Fancy and his boss, Bass, who Fancy had asked to make the transfer. What David got to in that scene was Fancy and Bass together reckoning with who would be living with the consequences of this cop going to Bed-Stuy, and it wasn't Fancy or Bass; it would be people in Bed-Stuy. What came out of Fancy thinking about that was him asking for the cop to be transferred to his precinct instead. Taking that on felt true to what we knew about Fancy as a character. What made the storyline work in the end wasn't Fancy making the right or wrong choice in any one scene, what's satisfying is the sequence of scenes. It keeps canceling itself out until finally what you're left with is people being themselves, being creatures of their past, coming to the present. It got to the truth that there are all kinds of inauthentic behaviors that masquerade as authentic, and destructive behaviors that masquerade as constructive. Every gesture is mixed with some complicating motivation. Sometimes our effort to disentangle those motives is an attempt to make things too simple—"I want to like that guy or I don't, but I don't want to have to feel that he has all these different things going on inside him." It's the business of writing to get all the things that are spinning inside a person going at once, because then what you wind up with is that irreducible obstinate finality of a human being. Four hundred years ago, Black people were brought here in chains and that failure of respect for the humanity of one group of people by another, the consequences of that act, are felt now in every life in this country, and will be felt for another four hundred years. That fact informs every scene, for the characters and the audience, whether they're aware of it or not, so the question is what you do with that. There cohabit in each of us elements of resiliency and elements of woundedness and imprisonment. What you don't do is try to hide from the complexity of your own feelings. Everyone in that story is marked by their own particular experience and their own particular weaknesses. You work with your eyes, and you try not to blink, and you listen, and you try not to turn away from all the different complexities of feeling. You let yourself feel all of the contradictions, and if you are able to render a world in sufficient complexity, then it all gets told.

After writing all that, David said he was glad, and that he knew he'd grown as a writer doing those additional scenes. The enormous opportunity that storytelling offers is the chance to accommodate all of the elements of one's own spirit and bring them into the present, into a moment where they're all kind of alive and interacting with one another, and in being alive and interacting they become healthier. That's the opportunity that Fancy gets, or chooses, by bringing the guy into his own station house. He gets to come to the present more fully, he gets to live into a future with this guy and with himself. It was one of the blessings of my life that David and I got to do that together too, even if not as much or as long as I would have liked.

David Mills wrote nine episodes for our show and "Taillight" was actually the last one before he left to go work on *ER*. He won a Humanitas Prize for the episode. He'd go on to work on *The Corner* and *The Wire* and *Treme* and won well-deserved recognition and awards for that work too. David Simon was able to give him things I couldn't, to allow him to live more freely in the work than I ever finally could, due to both my defects of character and David Simon's gifts of spirit. It's also probably fair to say that because more of the main characters in those shows were Black, instead of just, say, the lieutenant, each one had more freedom to be fully themselves both in the world of the show and in the imaginations of every writer who worked on those shows. David Mills died in 2010 at forty-eight of a brain aneurysm and he was one of the best writers to ever work in our medium.

* * *

The set on *NYPD Blue*—that was a pretty good set, especially once Jimmy Smits came. What Mark Tinker, Paris Barclay, and our production manager Bob Doherty fostered was a sense that everyone here knows what you're doing is important, and we know you know how to do it. We knew that the guy who was working the dolly grip was part of making the music. So each person was able to come out of themselves a little bit and acknowledge that they cared a lot about what was happening. Keep in mind that one episode was being shot while the following one was being planned. I was late all the time with the writing because I was changing it and thinking about it. I was seeing something in the editing room that made me want to write a new scene. They let me. One of the fortunate tricks of working like that was that no one could give us notes. The network didn't have a chance to say anything because they never got to read or see anything, and I think that's part of why Steven was okay with it. The other part was that the show was a hit and making a lot of people a lot of money. In those circumstances people are more willing to forgive late script delivery. And the work was good. Steven knew the work was good, and the other writers, the producers, and the actors knew the work was good. But it still messed with their daily lives. No one knew what their schedule would be, not what hours or even what days. Everyone just had to be available all the time. That's what I asked of them, but that's what I was giving too. It was just how I ended up working, how the writing happened. People had to have a lot of respect for one another to do things that way, a lot of trust. Part of the honor of working with the people that I worked with was I knew what they could do and they knew what I could do. It was fun. We got to create a world. And we did it by everybody bringing their imaginations to bear on creating that reality. That is no bullshit. I didn't think of the stairs in the station house. I didn't think of the way people were dressed. But all of it together made a world.

I started doing these raffles every Friday to end the week, which I'd keep doing on most of my shows. I'd bring a bunch of cash, usually from the track, a few thousand dollars, or more than a few, and we'd pull names out of a hat, extra hundred for some people, five hundred for someone else, a grand. End of the season raffles were even bigger. Other days I'd buy a hundred scratcher lotto tickets and give them out to people. I knew I put people through a lot, so it was another way to show my appreciation or try to make recompense. Plus, I'm wacky about money.

There was a lot of friendship, a lot of history. Of course Steven and I had known each other a while. Mark Tinker, my dear friend Billy Finkelstein, Walon Green—we'd all known one another twenty years by then, and now Bill Clark with us. We had bikes on the lot with our names on them, and we'd ride our bikes from the production office to the set to the commissary for lunch. One of us would shout, "Take the ramp!" and we'd all go left to the ramp, like kids. To be with friends and get to do work you're proud of, to all be working hard together, that's the best it gets.

We had such a good thing going and we wanted more. Capitalism asks us to want that too, and who are we to say no. The group of us started working on more shows together in various combinations, *Brooklyn South* and *Total Security*. We were lucky and unlucky enough that they both got picked up. The blessing of that delay we had on *NYPD Blue*, where I had an extra year to figure out the world and characters, we didn't get that this time. It was all so fast, and we had *NYPD* going. The networks were still very much locked into the twenty-two-episode season model then, and the pace of that work was just relentless. *Total Security* got canceled pretty quick, but *Brooklyn South* aired the full season; so between that and the fifth season of *NYPD*, I worked on forty-four hours of television in a single year. That's too much.

In part because it was on a different network, *Brooklyn South* was shot on a different lot, one that happened to be across town. So we were fucked. By the time I would get to set, I was inevitably pissed off because I had just spent an hour in traffic, and I knew I was failing the show. The kind of shows that we did required real hands-on participation by the writers and the producers, and it was just too tough. I couldn't get over there, and when I could get there I was mad and it just wasn't gonna happen.

I was slipping back into bad habits. Some of the positive developments from my heart problems were getting distorted again. Red wine can be good for your heart. I had started drinking a bottle or two a night. I knew I had to exercise, but my back and hips were hurting all the time, but I *had to* exercise, so I started taking Vicodin for the pain. I started taking fifteen Vicodin at a time for the pain. I was swinging from manic to depressed. I didn't have time to talk through episodes or beats with other writers, so I was just rewriting everything myself whenever I finally got to it and yelling at my friends. Rita and I started a nightly ritual with the kids called the egg-throwing ceremony. We'd each get an egg and all go face the vine-covered wall of the guesthouse and say something from the day that pissed us off and then throw that fucking egg against that fucking wall. I do recommend this if you have an available wall. It helped.

There was an episode of *NYPD* in the middle of that fifth season and Ted Mann was working on it. In the first season of our show he had done a script about a guy who thought he was a werewolf, Lou the werewolf (Dan Hedaya played him and he was exceptional). It was a strong episode, and there was an effective interrogation sequence, and Ted wanted to do another story about Lou the werewolf. For me at that time, anyone who wanted to do anything was okay with me as long as I didn't have to think about it, because we were so completely under the gun.

The script came in, and though it wasn't particularly effective yet, there was a moment in it that became the jumping-off point for us to start reworking it. This guy who thought he was a werewolf lived in the park (as a wolf he wouldn't be living in a co-op), and he saw a father abusing his son. That situation was one I felt would be good for a story. The JonBenét Ramsey case was also very much in the news then. I didn't have the vaguest idea then what went on inside the Ramsey house, nor do I now, but that too had engaged my imagination. A news story like that gets people speculating about a lot of different possibilities, and usually we think of wealth as a kind of protection against horror. So I was thinking about how such a thing could happen. Those things were bubbling around as I entered into working on this story.

Then I started thinking about my friend Israel. Near the gym where I worked out there was a homeless man I would see every day driving home, a big guy, Black. That was Israel. I would stop and talk with him, and he would answer by pointing to the Bible. He was mute. On Sundays I would take my kids with me, because it was family day at the gym, and afterward we would take him a meal. Once, maybe a year or so in, I tried to bring him new clothes, but he wasn't comfortable with that, and not too much time later he disappeared (attempted gestures of kindness are better predicated on an acceptance of the reality of the other person, but that's never been my strong suit).

As I began thinking about Ted's story and the father—assuming that a father had hurt his child and he was an intelligent person, and this had been going on for a while—how would he attempt to try to deflect suspicion away from himself? In the story he tries to pin it on the homeless guy, who had started as Lou but became Israel. As I was working on it, the mother began taking on more life as well. What was her part? What did she know or not know?

I was exhausted but this story started to feel different. The drama of this story was going to be found in very small moments, in very small gestures, as this multiple tragedy unfolds. Usually one of our episodes would start with a little personal business from one of the detectives that might help set up an episode's themes. But in this one, the first thing that you see is not one of our characters but the husband and wife. There's a dual movement going on there. On one hand, the drama is pushed very much to the foreground, the viewer is taken by the scruff of the neck and told this isn't going to wait, this is happening right now, but at the same time, it's happening very slowly. The viewer does not get any sort of wiggle room.

Simone invites those characters, the father and mother, Steve and Sherrie Egan, into the coffee room, and since there's no personal story going on, the only thing that our characters seem to be interested in is those two people—it's a kind of sensory deprivation.

"Some kind of refreshment?"

"No."

One by one, the audience is deprived of any kind of distraction within that scene except for attention to the behavior of those two people. Each time one of the characters declines any kind of stimulant, any kind of distraction, the cop notices, the cop looks up and takes that in. There's a second dramatist in that scene, the father, and the reason that all of these alternative distractions are eliminated is because the father is orchestrating what's going to happen. The father is saying, "Look at me, we are grieving parents, we are afraid something has happened" and he needs to get them to it, he needs to get them to the discovery of the son's body. He can't wait. The cops are aware that the interview is being orchestrated, even if the audience isn't. But they never tip that; they don't say anything about it until they walk out of the room.

The moment that the cops walk out, the chemistry changes completely. The audience is back with Simone and Sipowicz, in the absence of the characters who are outsiders to their world. Sipowicz confides a reaction that he did not exhibit in the presence of the strangers. His first words out of the coffee room are, "That guy talks too much, and he don't talk about the right things." That's a direct communication to the audience. To the extent Sipowicz is the surrogate for the viewer in dealing with those two characters, he's just identified the father as a killer, way early, way before any evidence comes in, but simply because in storytelling terms, that guy didn't do what he was supposed to do. What Sipowicz is saying is, "I know how a father is supposed to act when his son is missing. That guy didn't act that way, therefore his son isn't missing. His son's dead."

By jumping ahead of the facts, Sipowicz is expressing the divergence between epistemological truth, objectively verifiable truth, and the truth of storytelling. Every "fact" of the case, at least at the start, points to the guilt of the mute, points to the force in the story who has no voice. It's purely a matter of faith on the part of the surrogates for the audience, the detectives, that he didn't do it, because they know it's not the truth of this story.

When they do discover the body, they also discover that the boy has been sexually abused over a long period of time. As I was working on it, I began to feel it was important this story was told very, very slowly. I wasn't sure why, but I did. I didn't know where it was headed, but about halfway through I proposed to our directors, Steven DePaul and Paris Barclay, that this ought to be two episodes instead of one, even though we set up from the jump that the father did it. I didn't know what was going to be in the second episode, but I knew that the roots were going down. As long as you can feel that happening it's probably best to go on. And because of the extraordinary commitment and good spirit of our production unit we were able to make that adjustment, so we had "Lost Israel, Part One" and "Lost Israel, Part Two." Then it seemed to me Part Two was going to take a ninety-minute episode rather than a sixty-minute episode. That required going to the network, and that's one of the few instances in which it's good to be on a network whose ratings are diving, which ABC's were at that time, because they said, "Why not?"

Storytelling permits language to have its deepest, fullest expression, because it accommodates the dimension of time.

The way words and behavior accumulate, they take on more and new meaning, and that was happening in these episodes. Words are given that fuller dimension, and so too are the experiences of scenes as they accumulate one after another and modify the initial meaning that is experienced by the viewer when the scene is first rendered. Sipowicz, Simone, and Russell all become engaged in the case—Sipowicz with Israel, Simone with the father, and Russell with the mother, but in that division, they were working as one. All the scenes are connected, refracting back on one another. Very few scenes are played in which the following scene is not an effort to interpret what just transpired. And as this tragedy unfolds, as a boy is found dead, and you discover he had been abused, and then the mute Israel hangs himself, we're trying to figure out what it means along with the detectives. Sipowicz keeps going to the passages of the Bible that Israel had been pointing to, hoping they will explain, but they don't explain. The simple facts are inscrutable.

It is not easy work to be in the world of a tragedy. For an actor who is bringing everything they can to it, or a director, it's emotionally very taxing to stay in those feelings the way you have to to tell the story well. The actor Thom Gossom Jr. played Israel, Annie Corley and Brian Markinson played Sherrie and Steve Egan, and each of them gave all of themselves to this work. There's an expression in horse racing, "They didn't leave anything in the barn." That was true for every single person on that set helping us tell that story, but those actors in particular. They were ready to go wherever we needed to go. When that happens, it changes what you can do.

I discovered all sorts of things as I worked on those episodes. But they were hard things to discover, and it took time to get there. Even now, it's taking me time to tell this part. Every time

I've told the story of these episodes, it takes me nearly as long. In the second episode, the father eventually comes to Simone:

STEVE EGAN

I'm also going to confide something which I haven't to this point. In a sense it's my own burden and not specifically relevant to the case.

SIMONE

Please.

STEVE EGAN

When I was a child, I was abused myself.

SIMONE

Is that right?

STEVE EGAN

I'm not sure if you can understand the way that compounds my reaction to what's happened now thirty years later.

SIMONE

It has to make it that much more horrible.

STEVE EGAN

I haven't confided because I didn't want to burden Sherrie with it, with everything else she's dealing with.

SIMONE

Making it an extra burden that you're carrying around.

STEVE EGAN

So when I see this Detective Russell lavishing all this attention and time on my wife with these nonsensical theories.

SIMONE

Mr. Egan, I respect your concern for your wife, but I gotta tell you what I'm looking at, and that is someone that's in pain, who needs a little attention of his own.

STEVE EGAN

I don't know about needing attention, but I am in pain. I mean, I know what my son was going through. I know what it was like for him.
(sobs)

Oh God.

SIMONE

Steve, can I get you some water?

Steve shakes his head no.

STEVE EGAN

I was six years old, sent away to a sleepaway camp. I was fourteen months younger than any other kid there. Lie there at night in my bunk so homesick I couldn't stop crying. And I was a bed-wetter.

SIMONE

I was too.

STEVE EGAN

You were?

SIMONE

(nods)

I think a lot more kids are than people know.

STEVE EGAN

So I'd be lying there, homesick and humiliated, and
one night, Uncle Gil was on night duty. They called
all the counselors uncle. And he heard me crying. Or
maybe he saw my covers move when he shined his
flashlight because I would put the covers over my
head when I cried. And after a while, he would take
my hand, and put it between his legs. I didn't know
what it was about. I didn't know what he was doing.
All I knew was how homesick I was and he was the
only one who helped me and I was too afraid to say
that I didn't like it.

SIMONE

I'm sorry.

STEVE EGAN

Yeah. You live with what you live with. I mean those
were the cards I was dealt.

When someone admits to a cop that they were sexually abused
as a child, it's immediately considered a motive—it makes them
suspect. It's such a fundamentally corrupting experience that
can shape or distort the whole subsequent course of a person's
life. That story that's told by the father, that happened to me
and I had hidden it from myself. What I mentioned passingly
earlier in this book, the cards I was dealt—I had repressed the

whole thing. That's what happened, and I had never told anyone the full story before. Uncle Gil was the real guy at Camp Paradox. He was a very upstanding guy at the camp, and so he would come to the track in Saratoga too, my dad would invite him. He stayed at our house once after my first year of camp. It went on for years. I took that speech out and put it back in at least three times, the name even more times than that. The scene goes on:

STEVE EGAN

I don't know. I don't know if some things can be forgiven. How do you forgive a man who abuses a child's need and his trust?

SIMONE

I believe in forgiveness, Steve.

STEVE EGAN

You do?

SIMONE

Absolutely. Someone feels true remorse, I absolutely do.

STEVE EGAN

God that would be such a relief, to believe in forgiveness and protection.

SIMONE

For your son, for this man who abused you, for all of us. Everyone needs forgiveness. There's nobody who hasn't sinned.

STEVE EGAN

I'm grateful for you taking this time with me.

SIMONE

Whatever people say, we do this job because we
want to help. I'm grateful and honored that you'd
look to me.

In those scenes, and after, Simone believes he has no forgiveness in his heart, and that he's simply trying to move the father
to confess. Simone feels sick with comforting him even as he
knows that's what the father needs to give it up. As I tried to live
into this story it seemed to me that the only basis on which the
confession could be elicited from someone in such profound
despair, the radical despair of the soul, which is an absolute isolation from God, would be for someone to persuade him that
there was forgiveness. But as a dramatist it seemed to me that it
wouldn't be in any character, Simone or any other, to actually be
able to consciously forgive. All the time that I was working with
the Bible in that episode I was trying to figure out what the hell
I was doing with it. One of the ideas of a sacrament is that sometimes a priest is able to transmit something, which is separate
from the priest's own nature, to the person who receives the
sacrament. I felt that Simone was performing that function in
some sense, that his soul was possessed of a kind of forgiveness
that he himself didn't feel but that was able to elicit something
from the father, so that the father was finally able to confess.

SIMONE

You need to confront this, Steve. Keeping in mind the
forgiveness that we were talking about for everyone
involved.

STEVE EGAN

If you think I'll live under these conditions you're insane, where people think I'm some insane predatory monster, that's not going to happen, my friend.

SIMONE

There's forgiveness for everyone involved in this, Steve.

STEVE EGAN

I told you my plans, my friend, so please get out of my way.

Simone doesn't move; Steve's beginning to crack—

STEVE EGAN

I'm not prepared to dispute you are my friend, and I could use a friend very much. But at the same time you are a detective whose job is attributing guilt.

SIMONE

That is for lawyers and the courtroom. I am trying to understand what happened here.

STEVE EGAN

I thought you were trying to forgive everyone.

SIMONE

You know there's forgiveness. You know there's forgiveness. I need you to help me understand.

STEVE EGAN

Well, I'm exhausted, and I'm in a state of hopelessness.

SIMONE

That's all right. That's all right. Steve? You brought me here, and I need you to tell me why.

STEVE EGAN

Well, to receive these accusations, when so much of my life has been caring for Brian, when we were so close. And as much as I've been wounded and hurt, I tried to protect him from that, I tried to show him how much he was loved.

SIMONE

Were you physical showing your affection?

STEVE EGAN

Was I physical? We all want to be perfect parents and show our love in the perfect way, and at the same time we're human beings. And so which do you sacrifice? Do you stop trying to show your love at all if you can't show it in the perfect way? Do you stop being a parent to your only son and child? Believe me, for me to understand takes every fiber of asking God, to understand his forgiveness taking Brian and understanding His will.

SIMONE

So was it God who asked you to put Brian in heaven?

STEVE EGAN

I am not so presumptuous or egotistical to pretend I communicate with God. What I do know, is what's necessary for life not to become a grotesque insanity and to protect a child you love. I know the burden of what has to be done, because previously you can't forgive yourself, and you've beaten that in him. You can't forgive your own erection lying next to your counselor and you know you must be foul, and so you beat yourself in your boy. I don't presume to communicate with God, but can you believe in any God who didn't want his child protected when he sees him crying at night and wetting himself, and some monster, making him lie and hide and be so sad and afraid? How wouldn't God want him taken away?

(He shudders, opens wide and then closes his eyes—)

STEVE EGAN

Kill me, please. Please, shoot me in the head.

SIMONE

I can't.

STEVE

Help me confess. Hurry and get the pencil and paper.

If you try to stay true to the characters and to the situation, you ask yourself, is the behavior credible? And so to go back to the initial question that I started the work on the episode with, what would make a parent do this, I came to the answer that if a parent was hurting their child, abusing their own child in an ongoing way, I could understand believing it was better to do whatever felt necessary to end that ongoing hurt, even kill them, than keep hurting them.

The repetition of the word "forgiveness"—it can have twenty different meanings. It's an instrument of cynicism as uttered by Simone at the beginning. It's an instrument of corruption as first expressed by the father. And as the scenes go on and the context modifies, the word comes to have meanings beyond what the speaker intends. It's for that reason, because language can draw on all those different meanings as a result of context, that when you tell a story, parts of your unconscious and your preconscious come into play. As words collect and accumulate and create a context, they develop their own past, and we come to sense the different meaning of a word, say, "forgiveness," from what we felt it meant five minutes before, in a different scene.

One of the ways to discover forgiveness—I think one of the requirements—is the ability to draw the experiences of the past into consciousness so that your full soul can address them. When you try and think about things to write, what makes telling stories a useful enterprise requires a passion. It requires, in the nature of your engagement with the materials, a deep and genuine desire to render human experience in an important way. Then you have to stick with it, and not back down. Follow it out. I followed it out that time. And in doing that, the meaning of what happened to me changed. Storytelling is not therapy, but storytelling can be an instrument of healing in the sense of fulfilling the capacities of our humanity. So that was a sort of extra benefit that came to me.

When the episode aired, my mom happened to be staying with us. The next morning she told Rita that when they said the name Uncle Gil, she threw up. My mom and I never talked about it. When I talked to my brother about it since, he said none of them knew. My kids saw that episode, and they and Rita then carried that knowledge, and that had a not insignificant or straightforward impact on our family. I wasn't thinking about any of that when I wrote it. I was following the story. I was getting to the truth of these characters. I was honoring my collaborators by doing my best. I don't think I could have said what happened to me any other way.

* * *

Those episodes aired in December of 1997. It also happens to be true that in 1998 I started trying in earnest to get sober again. It would be too easy to say that bringing those memories to the surface is what allowed me to try to get sober, but it also makes sense that I couldn't get sober for real as long as there was a part of me committed to keeping that stuff hidden. But none of that was at the level of consciousness. What was at the level of consciousness was that my kids were getting older, in particular my boy Ben was twelve by then, and I was scared of the stuff that happened between my dad and me happening with him. It was to my daughters' great benefit that they were, in my mind, more safely my wife's province and so not as vulnerable to my weaknesses of spirit (not that they got out scotfree, they're captive in a different way, in the vast project of my care). But Ben, I was scared he'd use, or perhaps certain of it, and in some magic, selfish way I thought if I could get sober that would keep it from happening, or at least make me a fraction less of a bum and fraud when I tried to be his parent through that happening. To the extent that that was at the level of consciousness is a credit to my wife, like most other things. That was still a diseased interpretation of events, but it was one that had some benefits.

At the same time, Jimmy Smits let us know he would be leaving the show, and that his decision was somewhere between mostly and entirely due to my always delivering scripts so late. That was another sign that perhaps I needed to shift some habits (though in time we would all learn the scripts came no earlier when I was sober).

I did a three-day inpatient stay at St. John's Hospital to supervise my physical withdrawal. If you're taking enough stuff, kicking is not pretty; in fact, it's so terrifying and painful that at first you think you might die, and then you're certain you want to. Then the physical pain begins to remit, and what's left is all the other pain you have to figure out what to do with. To that end, this particular program had an extensive outpatient group therapy component, six months or so, including groups for partners and families that Rita took part in. I found myself in other rooms that people in recovery find themselves in. You get responsibilities in those rooms, you're on coffee or snacks or dessert, and I'd get very into my responsibilities. Huge spread from Whole Foods. Best fucking fruit plate the room had ever seen. The widest assortment of berries. In a lot of these rooms, I was a bit of an outlier in terms of financial success, including in the outpatient group I was in. The woman running that group, she was taken with me. I was very wise there. Sage Dave. I was lending people money. That looks like a generous act. In fact, it has an element in it of "look at me, I'm a rich guy." I'm a big tipper. The most normal situation I'm not going to let be a normal situation. I'm a rich guy. That's me, Dave the rich guy. I was inviting people from recovery to our house all the time. Sometimes they were in rough shape. Rita eventually asked me to meet people elsewhere. It didn't always feel safe. I was excited and ill-equipped, full of good intention and not packing the gear to communicate. The responsibility that you had was to be humble, but I wasn't. I was dry but not really sober.

At the outpatient program "graduation" I told a story about going to my children's rooms to say good night and tell them I love them. It's this circuit of three rooms and I did it every night. And I said, "The truth is, for a long time, most nights, I didn't feel anything. And I'd feel so alone for not feeling anything. Just deep despair. They're right there, we're saying the words and I can't feel anything. But I'd do it anyway. I kept going. And now, on some nights, I can feel my love for my children, and theirs for me in return." People who've spent some time in recovery might recognize this as a version of "fake it 'til you make it," and William James's idea that behavior guides feeling, not the other way around. That's true, but my kids were there for my graduation that night along with their mother. My not feeling anything when I told them I loved them, that was news to them, and that's a lot to ask children to understand. There was some truth to be shared with them in that story about my experience as their father, and how showing up even when you can't feel the reward is its own act of love, but I was also doing it for an audience.

The psychiatrist Carl Jung and a drunk exchanged a series of letters. The drunk reached out to Jung first, he asked if there was any way that he could save himself, because he knew that, the way he was going, was about to die. And Jung told this guy that he was a hopeless case, that he had seen people in that situation and there was nothing that medicine could do for them, that the only hope he had seen was a few people who had had a spiritual conversion. Those few people had been able to recover, but absent that, Jung saw no hope. Twenty years later, this fellow wrote to Jung and said, well, you know, I had a spiritual experience, and I got well, and I thought you might be interested. And this guy was one of the early guys involved in what became AA, Alcoholics Anonymous. He had been able to have a spiritual experience, by being with others and talking with others and feeling connection in that shared experience. Jung wrote him back, saying a very curious thing. He said that what he had been afraid to tell this guy at that time was his idea that drunks, addicts of any kind, were in fact souls that had been cut off from God and who were reaching out to complete themselves; that they were split selves, damaged selves, and in their damage were so unable to complete their natures as human that they were reaching out, that their addictive behavior was, in fact, a kind of crippled expression of their desire for God. Jung said that it had always interested him that the Latin for "soul," *spiritus*, was also the Latin for alcohol. In English, it's called "spirits." What Jung said in his letter was that the formulation he would propose was *spiritus contra spiritum*, the recovery of the soul to defeat the alcoholism.

I'd started teaching again, two weeks each summer in '97 and '98. A mix of college students and aspiring writers and working writers. The ones who needed housing I'd put up in apartments on my own dime. And I'd show them episodes and we'd talk about them. My writing process had already shifted by then so that I dictated everything, in those days to the wonderfully patient and helpful George Putnam (as a thank-you I named a serial killer after him), and so between that and writing on the set with actors, I was always writing in public. Working that way neutralized some of the obsessive-compulsive behavior I got into when I was writing alone. It was an audience, but it was also a fellowship of spirit. Both things can be true. Many things can be true. There's no healing all at once. I'm not done yet.

* * *

Jimmy Smits agreed to give us five episodes at the start of the sixth season. As with David Caruso, his departure was announced between seasons, and that became part of the storytelling challenge. The audience already knows this character is leaving, so how do you make them feel and experience that departure?

With the character John Kelly's departure, we embraced a certain amount of the audience's cynicism and disappointment in whatever mysterious institutions and behind-the-scenes dealings had brought that outcome about, and made it the Internal Affairs Bureau's machinations that so thoroughly dogged and alienated Kelly that he decided to leave. With Bobby Simone, I wanted to honor the connection the audience and the characters had developed over multiple years. If the character is leaving, that is an experienced death for the purposes of the dramatic structure. You'll get the most genuine junction of the viewer's experience if, at the level of story, he literally dies. But the audience was so saturated with the preexisting knowledge about Jimmy's plans to leave, it seemed to me that no storyline that relied on any sort of unprepared-for outcome would work. The practical result would be the audience going, "Okay, three episodes with regular stories, he's going to get hit by a bus or he's gonna be shot." They wouldn't be in it, so instead it needed to be slow, the drama would have to come from the realization of what was happening. I wanted it to feel like a real death, how things could really go wrong, all the emotional processes we go through to face a loss like that, and so I started talking to my brother Bob.

After my dad passed, my brother, who had also been a surgeon, retrained himself as a hospice physician to care for the terminally ill. He started and then ran a hospice in Buffalo. He became an expert on palliative care and established hospice programs in Romania, in Poland, in Hungary. He'd seen every kind of death, and every kind of grief. I choose to believe that my father, in his own inability to accept himself, was instrumental in teaching my brother that there was another way to be a physician. If you end the story at my dad's death, it's not the whole story. I believe that through his work, my brother put my dad at rest, and in the very sadness of his death, my dad made possible the comfort of many thousands of strangers.

As a society, we have enormous anxiety about medicine, and we bind our anxiety in different ways. One way is to idolize the doctors and nurses. *ER. House.* But then again anytime a person gets on a jury he tries to stick it to the quack. Those differences are all tied to how much power people do or don't feel. When people feel empowered, they let their hostility come out. When they don't feel empowered, they mythologize: "I love to watch them take care of people." Not long before we were working on this story I was on this panel with James Watson, one of the guys who won the Nobel Prize for discovering the structure of DNA. The Sloan Foundation was hosting the panel, and they had given me a grant to make a show that would humanize scientists, and I can't turn down money. I'm on this panel and I'm suggesting that there are these deep misgivings in the public consciousness about what people perceive as the devil's bargain that science has made, the sense that knowledge without understanding is a terrifying state of being. Watson seemed to me to only want to think of himself as a hero. This guy has tried to get four different movies made about himself. He thinks it's a casting issue, that more handsome actors should play scientists, there's no fundamental distrust. I point out that the fact that Frankenstein gets remade every decade would suggest maybe there is, people think the monster's out of control. He calls me a misfit from the Yale English department who is afraid of science's promise. I say, "In a way, that's it. I don't meet as many scientists who can meet my eyes in conversation as I do people who pump gas." I make friends everywhere I go.

For me as a kid, the hospital was a very, very, very frightening place. I always felt a little bit like an intruder because I had the feeling that that was where Dad did his important work and I was taking him away from that. There was a sense of separate agendas, of agendas in the hospital that didn't have to do with my emotional life. Bob had found his own way into that space, to be with our dad in medicine. Once I started having heart problems, I was bringing all of those old feelings into being a patient. Trying to be good for the doctors but feeling like their agenda wasn't mine. Bob was always very involved, talking with my doctors, explaining things to me and Rita, making sure I got the best care, but that was still a complicated feeling, for both of us. I wanted to show the process of being in a hospital from the point of view of the patient and family, to stay with it even as things go wrong, and to show the physicians as people as they are perceived by a patient.

As I worked on the story, I found myself calling my brother twice, three times a day. From the beginning of the sixth season, literally from the first scene in the first episode, I wanted to put into play emotionally that Simone was at risk. The very first scene is a dream, Simone with Patsy Ferrara (the wonderful Brad Sullivan), who taught Simone to fly pigeons. They're on the roof under a bright blue sky, Patsy is telling Simone to breathe deep. (In the third season Bobby had tried to take care of his old mentor as he struggled with dementia, but in his dreams Patsy's mind is clear as day.) What starts seeming like a bit of a chest cold turns into an infection that goes to his heart. I wanted to make sure the course of that infection, the treatment they give, the limits of what medical intervention could do all played. I was talking to my brother constantly, more than we'd talked since we were kids.

I asked Bob to come out to L.A. while we shot the hospital scenes. He helped me and the actors understand the states of mind of the characters and the physicians, of Simone, of Russell, and how different kinds of doctors deal with this process. What Bob helped me get to, what he knew and practiced was that the deepest responsibility of a medical practitioner is not curative, it's pastoral. "I will walk with you into whatever darkness may come." What does that look like? David Barrera played the young Dr. Carreras, and the first night Simone and Russell are there he says to Russell, "If you want to eat here the nurses can have an extra dinner delivered, just fill out a second menu at the desk." But not every doctor is like that, and so between the two doctors, Carreras and Swan, we dramatize that distinction. The surgeon, Dr. Swan, keeps insisting on the possibilities of science, of going a step further, and one would think that's hope. But Russell hates him because he's talking down, he's trying to keep the science a mystery only he knows. Dr. Carreras is the one who instead starts opening the door to the possibility that Bobby may not get better, and who finally explains there are worse things than dying. He walks with them and in walking with them makes them brave enough to complete the journey. When Bob was building the hospice in Buffalo, he had them design it as a circle, so pacing family members could never get lost. It's letting your imagination be with people. Getting to work on those episodes, it was a chance for my brother and me to be together in a different way. We weren't just split parts of my dad, we were a unity. For maybe the first time since we were little, we were walking together again.

The fifth episode is a living into acceptance. I wanted to make that available to the audience as well. And I wanted to honor Jimmy Smits. He gives his whole body to those episodes, his whole spirit. The great actors are all storytellers. Their particular gift is that their entire being is their instrument. It's indistinguishable the way an actor moves, the way he blinks, it's all a oneness and a presence. As a writer, you feel like you're stealing, you just get shivers because the artist is so present. He or she so embodies not only the character but the moment. That's why being on the set for the moment of art is kind of a religious experience. The episode ends with Bobby dreaming of Patsy and his birds. Patsy is preparing him to go, and what Brad Sullivan who plays Patsy is doing is making it poetry ("Now, if a bird goes over the horizon, does it continue to fly, grow, and change? Even in a strange place, and a bird disappears, isn't it going home and to be okay, for example?"). While that's happening, all of the characters are coming to say goodbye to Bobby in his hospital bed. When Patsy brings the son that Bobby and Diane lost to hold his hand in his dream ("You're going to see your boy constantly"), the audience sees Sipowicz holding Bobby's hand and promising to walk with Diane through what's to come ("I'll take care of her"). The man who raised Bobby says to him, "Now I take it you've grown, and I can leave you on your own," and the reason that moves the audience is because the audience has grown emotionally in their own experience of accepting this loss. Every person on that set was crying when we shot that episode. Paris Barclay directed it, and we had to move the camera setups and monitors farther away than usual, because we were all crying. Letting yourself feel a loss, bringing grief fully into the light—we don't often let ourselves do it, but it's a privilege to be a part of.

We shot those episodes in the fall and my family went on a trip to New York for the holidays that year. When we got back it was New Year's Day and I was exhausted. But I couldn't let myself rest, or be with my family, and then I was sick with myself because I couldn't rest or be with my family. So I went into the office. Miserable. I started putting my hand in the couch, feeling under the cushions. I found some Vicodin and I took it and I hated myself so much. And that was the actual last time I used. January 1, 1999. Fifty-three years old.

* * *

The next year, our seventh season, was the end of my contract on *NYPD Blue*. I decided it was time for me to move on too. Rick Schroder had joined the cast in the sixth season and he was well settled in. Steven and Bill and Mark, they agreed it was the right time to make the change. I was late with pages all the time, and I think everyone was more than a little ready to figure out what the show and working on the show could feel like without me running it. I was changing lines on set, moving words around, adding whole speeches; the actors had taken to writing down their line changes on nearby props. The language was getting more inverted, which could make it harder to remember.

Rita decided it was important to memorialize those last weeks on *NYPD Blue*, so she and a distant cousin of mine named Marc Ostrick made a documentary they ended up calling *Without a Net*. At one point Bill is asking me which character is going to die in the finale, the culmination of the season's ongoing storyline, which also has a fair number of implications for the hundreds of people who work on the show. "I don't fucking know, Bill. If I knew who the fuck was going to die, I'd tell you." There's a moment when you see Kim Delaney waiting outside her trailer with her ten-year-old son Jack, and Jack tells the camera, "We're waiting for pages." Toward the end I'm sitting in front of the soundstage with a bunch of the actors, Rick and James McDaniel and Kim and Andrea Thompson. I think we were waiting for them to reset the stage based on some changes I'd just made. I've got some bananas for a snack and I say, "You know what, throw it at me." I break some off a piece of banana and hand it to Rick and he pelts me one and starts to laugh. Then he passes the banana and each of the actors gets a throw in, they're all laughing. I say, "It feels good, doesn't it?"

The actor Scott Cohen was recurring that season, doing great work as a crooked cop, and I gave him some real strange lines to say. At one point he's getting ready to shoot and I'm saying to him, "Lose 'that.'" "What?" "'That,' lose the word 'that.'" I was so focused on the meter of things. When I finally watched the film Rita and Marc made I said, "That's not a documentary, that's an intervention."

In the middle of shooting that season, the Humanitas Prize comes back around. Jimmy's last episode, "Hearts and Souls," wins. I was still pretty new in sobriety. And the whole time during the ceremony I'm looking at Father Kieser and I'm thinking how I had always hated this guy, how he would look at you and smile with his buckteeth and his close-set eyes, and that night I'm noticing he's got a bit of amblyopia going too, a lazy eye. I'm thinking when I get up there I'm going to call him out. So I get up and I'm looking at Father Kieser, who's right next to the podium, and I say, "I've never liked Father Kieser. In particular, I have taken offense at this smile which is chronically on his features, and which he evinces even now as I speak. It's like he's saying he knew something about me that I didn't know about myself. But recently I have been relieved of certain obsessions. I thank God that I have lived long enough to have come to understand that that darkness in which I believed I must move, and in which my characters must live, is in fact cast by God's sheltering hand. And that's what Father Kieser knew about me that I didn't know about myself."

None of that was what I planned to say. I had planned to say I suspected him of child abuse. The idea that we understand

and control what we're doing, and therefore ought to have a plan and guide our steps accordingly—of all my gratitude I am most grateful to have been relieved of that sense of necessity.

A month or so later Father Kieser called me and said, "I'm dying. Would you come and sit with me?" And I did. It turned out he'd been quite ill at the time of that dinner and in fact his amblyopia was a manifestation of a brain tumor. As I sat with him, sometimes he was delirious, and he kept saying to me, "You must write about Paul. You must write about Paul."

5.

Turn Me Loose

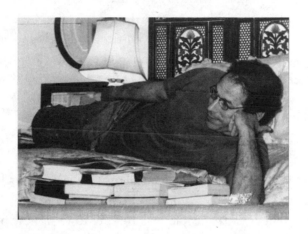

HERE'S A LITTLE STORY about Hollywood. When I left *NYPD Blue*, I said to my agent, "Okay, go get me a deal. I'll work for anybody but Les Moonves." The experience with him on *Brooklyn South*—I didn't love that. He seemed to me to think he was the only one who understood how the world worked, and he didn't. He also had an active disdain for artistic ambition—treated it as a self-delusion, which maybe it is, but the forced ironic pose, I can't work like that. My agent goes out, gets me a development deal with Paramount, we sign it. A week later, he calls back, "Uh, Les Moonves is now in charge of Paramount." So now I've got to pitch this guy I hate. I don't think he liked me very much either.

One pilot I wrote for UPN was this show *John From Else-where and His Friend Tex*. It was UPN so it was about younger people. Imagine aliens come down and want to save the spe-cies, maybe they'd visit some junkies. It was kind of like a com-plement to *Buffy the Vampire Slayer*, which I knew about and appreciated because my kids watched it. I liked that it was doing a number of things at once. I was imagining fuckups like I'd been, real messes. Aliens and hustlers and skels and addicts in New York, a whole show with just the junkies and snitches and creeps who were usually my favorite characters to write. There was a character named Zenon of Nyack. They passed on it.

I'm chastened, so I started working on something a bit closer to what I'm known for. More cops in New York, but I wanted to complicate it. Once or twice Bill or friends of his had been pulled into a task force with the FBI. The intricacies of that— the different agendas people are working toward, how people withhold information from one another—I thought could make for some good storytelling. Thematically, what that dra-matizes is the difference between information and understand-ing. Technology was shifting the way cops and the FBI did surveillance, the same way it was shifting the way the rest of us did everything. There was so much more information to obtain so much more easily, but that information doesn't necessarily translate to understanding. In fact, that onslaught of informa-tion can in its own way be isolating—we don't know what to do with the information, we become nervous about what can be shared and what can't, we don't know who to trust. I wanted to tell a story of people struggling with that and figuring out how to live in a world like that. I called the show *Big Apple*, and it was about New York, but really it was the Tree of Knowledge of Good and Evil in the garden. Everyone in this show has taken a bite, and they're trying to figure out what to do with the information they now have, same as Adam and Eve.

The NYPD detectives would be the audience's surrogates in the story. At least initially, much of our understanding would be tied to theirs. But while *NYPD Blue* was a story with two leads who we knew were the center of our focus, this show would push beyond that. One arc would be about the detectives coming to accept that they were becoming a part of a larger organization, and, with that, for the audience to accept that every character was important.

So I go in and pitch this show—surveillance and the garden and all of it. Les hears the pitch and he says, "Oh, that's great. I think I understood about thirty percent of that."

"And is that high or low for you?" I say.

"Let's shoot in seven weeks."

That's where the record scratch goes. I don't usually work that fast. Something doesn't feel right. But I don't say no to getting to work.

* * *

There was a restaurant on Wilshire, near 26th Street, Drago, that was a three-minute drive from our house then. It was one of three restaurants I'd just about ever go to, and being it was closest to my house, I'd go there probably once a week during *NYPD*, with Bill or Bill and cops or Bill and Rita or Bill and Rita and the kids. We ate early, and when we'd be leaving we'd usually see Ed O'Neill coming in. I'd learn later it was after they finished the *Married . . . with Children* taping each week. He'd come in a lot of times by himself and have a glass of wine and dinner, and what you noticed was a person at peace with himself, able to enjoy himself and take his time. Since those things eluded me, I was fascinated by that. I'd watch him and he was so different from Al Bundy. He's a big guy, a former football player, but he moved through the room with a kind of warmth and softness and grace. I'd think to myself, "This guy is a great fucking actor, because he's nothing like that guy." We'd see each other enough that we started nodding when we passed, then saying, "Hello, Ed," "Hello, David." At least two years, just saying hi.

As I'm working, quickly, on this new script, I realize I want him to play the lead, Detective Mooney. I get the script sent to his agent so they can both read it. Something gets lost in translation and they read it thinking I want him to play Maddock, who's this Irish gangster (who Michael Madsen would do wonderful work with). We meet to talk about the show and we're having a meal together for the first time and I ask what he thinks.

"Have you read the script?"

"Yeah, it's wonderful."

"Well, I want you to do the role."

"Great, I always wanted to play a Westie."

"What are you talking about?"

"The role. The guy. The Westie."

"No, Ed, I want you to play the cop. Mike."

"Mike? David, honestly, I wasn't reading it for that role. I was reading it for the other guy. I'd have to read it again."

"Well, it's the lead."

"Okay. Well, I'm probably gonna do it. But why do you want me to do it? Why me?"

"I just have a feeling about it. The restaurant. I like the way you carry yourself."

This was only two years after *Married . . . with Children* had ended. Eddie has said since then that this was the moment he realized he was gonna have a career after that show. Then once he saw the work he was doing, that was when he realized he really could act as well as anybody. And he can. Think of having a gift and never being sure if you'll get to share it again. It's terrifying.

Stanley Kunitz has a poem that says, "In a murderous time / the heart breaks and breaks / and lives by breaking." I've learned that's true for us all but it's especially true for actors. To do what they do, to feel compelled to give oneself to expressing other lives and feelings, and then to put themselves at risk, constantly, of rejection or belittlement—to be at the mercy of others just to get to do what they feel called to do. That's incredibly beautiful. It's sacred. And each of them knows they're lucky if they ever get one great part, or one big part that gives them a living, but those big parts can feel like a kind of trap too. I've always loved giving people who've had a part like that another time at bat. They're so happy to be in the world again and they show up. I believe we all deserve that chance. The other thing about it is the audience brings all sorts of thoughts and feelings to meeting an actor like that again in a new form, and most of those thoughts and feelings they're not even aware of. Because I believe that's how most of us go about meeting people in our lives, you can get something as an artist by tapping into that on purpose.

We had to hurry. Seven weeks is nothing. It's no time at all, especially for casting an ensemble show with a thirteen-episode commitment, but we got lucky. Michael Madsen and David Strathairn joined up along with Eddie, Glynn Turman, and Dylan Baker, who was in that cast in a guest role. Titus Welliver had a recurring role as a doctor on *NYPD Blue* and was in the main cast on *Brooklyn South* and I knew I wanted him to play Jimmy Flynn, an FBI guy who was in over his head. Donnie Wahlberg at that point was still known as a member of that boy band, but he had done a remarkable scene in *The Sixth Sense* and we got him to play one of Maddock's guys whose girlfriend gets murdered in the first episode, which kicks the whole story off.

We didn't yet have our female lead, Sarah Day, who's brought to New York from the Denver office to bring some fresh eyes and figure out if someone's been compromised. You needed someone you could watch watching the world, someone who could model a faith that it was okay not to understand everything at once and that you'd come to understand eventually. The casting director showed me the reel for an actress named Kim Dickens. She was in this movie called *Things Behind the Sun* where she was a singer who had a song about being raped when she was a teenager. The song's becoming popular and a journalist who knew her then starts covering the story. There was just so much going on in her eyes that once I saw the reel I said, "That's our girl." They said, "Yeah, we think she's great too, but her agent says she doesn't want to do TV." I said, "See if she'll meet with me so I can try to convince her." And she was willing, so she came to the office and we talked some about the part but mostly I talked to her about what I saw in her work, what she was bringing to it. Afterward she called her agent and said she'd do the show. Good people want to be seen, and when good people feel seen, it makes them brave.

We wanted to shoot on location in New York, but I didn't really think through the implications of that for my family (historically never a strength of mine). Elizabeth and Ben were in high school then and Olivia was in middle school, so it was not a period where they could just switch schools or bolt for a month or two, and Rita wasn't going to leave them unsupervised either. So I ended up living by myself in the Regency Hotel while we were shooting. Rita came with me the first week and put real sheets and quilts from home in my hotel room, but I missed my family a whole lot. Henry Winkler was doing a play then so he was staying at the same hotel and I think he could tell I was lonely, or maybe he was too, and we started having meals together. We had never really known each other even though we lived pretty close in L.A. and our kids went to school together. He'd gone to drama school at Yale. We'd talk about New Haven and our work and our families. I wrote him a part as a lawyer in some of the later episodes of the show, and he was so funny and weaselly and pathetic and great in the role. We became good friends. We stayed friendly when we got back to L.A., but in those months he might have saved my life. I don't know what I would have gotten up to alone if I hadn't made a friend like Henry then.

* * *

Even though I was sad most of the time I was back in my room, there was such good work happening. And there was a kind of blessed collaboration with all the actors on that show, but especially Eddie. If I go in to pitch a show and a network executive asks, "Well, what's the guy's background?" I say, "I don't know. I know what his present situation is and depending on how things go, we'll see what his past was." I'm not being withholding or clever. When you start to develop a relationship with a character, a situation, or a plot, there's a kind of respect that requires an acceptance of the relative inaccessibility of the character's past, that is, a sense of awe, of mystery. I can trust myself to know how a character will behave in a particular situation, but I don't know the lived facts of his past experience until I watch that behavior and then, in a constructive relationship with an actor, infer what the character's past must have been. After we got the show started, Eddie and I were trying to figure out why Mooney was such an isolate. All of his relation-

ships were confined to the professional sphere, so we were trying to figure out what his personal life must have been like. We
started to improvise a situation with his sister, imagining he
had a sister who needed care.

We don't meet the sister until the third episode of the show.
We brought on Brooke Smith, another extraordinary actor
who was associated with a particular role (she was the kid-
napped girl in the pit in *The Silence of the Lambs*) to play Lois,
Mike's sister, who we figured out was dying of Lou Gehrig's
disease. I was desperate to get the details right. It was precious
to me that every fold of the bed be right, to know how his sister
would have sat in the yard and waited for the kids to go by. I've
never been willing to do the exposition that would facilitate the
viewers' understanding of a character's past unless the dialogue
would occur naturally within the scene. The only sense that
you get during that episode of what her past was is one line,
when Mike says to her, "The lives you change teaching," talking about the girls who now take care of her as she's dying.
That's as much as he would have said, even if it's a little cryptic.

There's a lot of business about the blender. He thinks if he
can figure out the right blender, she'll stay alive. She's only
sticking around trying to figure out a way that he's going to be
able to live after she's gone. She's trying to prepare him for the
fact that she's going to stop eating. The way Lou Gehrig's disease works is first you can't swallow, and then you can't
breathe—if you don't die of inanition, which is a lack of nutri-
tion, then you finally die of suffocation, and she doesn't want
that.

My prejudice as a writer was always to stick with the quotidian, the nuts and bolts, the daily stuff of life. It was probably out
of fear, out of not trusting deeper emotions. That's a kind of
savage way, a primitive way of working. The scenes with Mike

and Lois, they started to bring this whole other sense of feeling to the show. If you stick with the characters and their situations, the natural impulse of those characters' spirits, over the course of time, is going to lead them into what is other than quotidian.

We did a scene that culminated with Mike playing the harmonica for her because Ed can really play. This is what I mean about a blessed collaboration with other artists. After we had done that sequence, Ed came to me and said he had been to the Hayden Planetarium on his day off, and there was a person sitting next to him who had Lou Gehrig's disease. Immediately we started thinking, "Would that be something that Mike would try, as part of his denial process?" I think Mooney held as his trump card, "Well, if I haven't taken her to the Hayden Planetarium yet, she's not going to die, because we still have that to do." When he sees that she's failing, he realizes now's the time.

And so he calls in his favors as a cop, arranges an escort, and they travel across the city to go to the planetarium. We got permission to shoot in the Hayden Planetarium. The logistics of something like that are just enormous and typically take weeks, but we had two hours' advance notice and everybody worked so hard. I remember, there was a kid I'd known for a long time, through a decade when neither of us drew a sober breath. He had been very ill and thank God he was spared; he was a set decorator or some damn thing, forgive me for not knowing exactly. We were getting Lois ready to go, and it certainly was not his job, but he came up to me and whispered, "You better put a line in about the snow because I think there's snow coming." And when everyone cares that much about a production, it's so much fun.

Then the snowstorm came. The drivers, I remember, were

working so hard to get us across town and to get us in, and the director of photography risked his life to be up as high as he was to get this shot of the police escort to the planetarium in the snow, the red and blue lights through the white. The DP went up in the air and there wasn't an instant's doubt—the story is always a person laying his body down for somebody else, one or another version of that. It's the way we transcend the illusion that we are separate. That's the gift of this peculiar signifying brain that we have.

When you've done your job as a writer, you properly disappear. In that scene, we moved beyond the blessed ordinariness of things. We had earned the right to tell that part of the story. When Mike and Lois are starting on their trip out in the universe, you just watch them watching the stars. The only dialogue you needed in that scene was, "Thank you, Michael." "Thank you, sis." Because you've made your journey with them, and you know everything that's in their hearts. It would be an impiety, it would be a different kind of sentimentality, to have them say more at that point.

It's absolutely the best part of it, to be with brothers and sisters in a shared enterprise. For us as artists, that's as good as life gets. And that can happen even in something that's a doomed operation from the beginning, with all sorts of arcane politics at play.

My concerns with the boss redoubled once the show was getting scheduled. Les decided to put the show up against *ER*, after *Survivor*, which could be interpreted as a compliment but in its own way was a death sentence. The audience that might like our show the most already has appointment viewing on our competitor, and the audience who is tuned in to our channel just wants to be told who's getting voted off the island. The things you can't control you have to let go of. We just tried to hit the ball straight, we tried to do the best we could every day. We got great reviews. People loved Eddie. But not enough people watched. We were canceled after five weeks. We shot eight episodes and they didn't even air the last three.

I had DVDs pressed to send to the actors so they could at least see the work they did (one of the dogs got the corner of my copy). The front cover was a painting Rita had done that I had wanted to be the show art but the network rejected, and on the back there was an image of a handwritten note thanking them for their work. The commitment of everyone involved was just amazing, it made me so grateful to be doing the work that I was doing. That's one I wish more people could see. I loved that show.

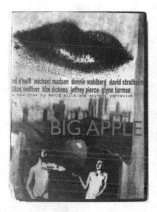 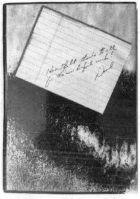

* * *

I learned late in life to obey my wife's commands without question, but even though I learned I only do it intermittently. I live in terror of her judgments but I rarely take the next step of following her instructions. In my consciousness my wife is a brooding, metaphysical omnipresence who has saved my life.

She knew I wanted to find a different kind of story to tell, and she would change the environment around me to help me tell it. My Paramount deal was still going and we were living large. We started renting an apartment in New York (I didn't want to have to live in a hotel again, and the kids were about to start heading East for college). We flew private so we could take our dogs with us. The other thing my wife would do is put books everywhere, scatter them around in our bedroom, stacks next to every toilet, and then she'd come back a few days later and take inventory, "Oh, he seems to have read some of this, we'll put more on this subject in here . . . He didn't like this, we'll take this out." There was a feeling between us that I was moving into a new phase. I was much more in the world of books and ideas and stories than my life. Rita and the kids seemed to understand that they would have to come with me into the work if they were going to be with me at all, and even then they would have to accept a fair bit of distance. They journeyed as much as they could. It's like you're playing the big game, get on a run down the field, and the people who love you are running alongside and cheering you on, giving you their energy, and eventually they have to stop and just watch you go. I don't know which one of us remembered Father Kieser's directive first, but after *Big Apple* was canceled, when I was back home in L.A. in the spring and then on Martha's Vineyard in the summer, I was rereading the Bible a lot, and books about St. Paul started proliferating around the house.

He was called Saul of Tarsus before he was Paul. Tarsus was under the control of Romans, and the Romans had this brilliant administrative idea which was that in areas they conquered, they gave the people citizenship to give them a little stake in things (an example we might have considered emulating). In Judaism, as it existed in the time of Christ, there were two dominant schools. The Sadducees, the priestly caste, believed in the books of Moses as sort of the whole game—they took care of business. Jerusalem was the center of the temple, and that's where the Sadducees were, and they were the bosses. Then there was another group called the Pharisees, who believed that you could try and figure out the book, how the book and the prophetic utterances applied, and they founded synagogues, separate houses of worship, and they weren't so tied to the big temple in Jerusalem.

Saul shows up in Jerusalem. In the New Testament, it's said that Saul was a Pharisee. But there's been discussion of certain evidence within the document that suggests he was something else, not really a Sadducee, but a tough guy, an enforcer. The reason for that speculation is that he was responsible for the murder of one of Christ's apostles, the stoning of St. Stephen.

The way that came about was that Saul was an outsider. He came from a different colony and we don't know what his situation was in Jerusalem, but he wasn't in the inner circle. He never met Christ. After Christ was crucified and whatever happened three days later, the followers, the disciples of Christ, began to circulate the story that this guy was the Messiah and he had risen, and Saul felt left out.

I remember once I was sitting in a library at Yale, during that year or more when I would write the same twelve pages word for word every day. Every morning praying that that would be the day I would be able to change at least one word. Couldn't do it. Couldn't pay for my electricity, couldn't do anything. I remember sitting in the library and the world was going on, some guy was buying a Reese's Cup and somebody else was talking, and I was thinking, "I'm never going to be a part of anything. I just don't know how to do it."

So I can imagine somebody in Jerusalem, hearing people talk, "Oh, seems like maybe the Messiah just came, and maybe he was resurrected too." This guy, trying to get in among the priests, in the library, watching 'em buy the Reese's Cups, thinking, "How do I get to be part of it?" There are all kinds of ways. One way is to say, "Hey, if these people say that was the Messiah, how come we're still walking around? If he isn't the Messiah, then they're blasphemers. If they're blasphemers, terrible is the wrath of God. Let us fuck them up." And so Saul organized a group and they stoned St. Stephen to death.

He finally had a way in, and he goes to the head of the Sadducees and says, "I'm the guy who fucked up St. Stephen. Turn me loose." And the high priest says, "Go to Damascus and fuck 'em up there." So he leaves.

There he was on the road to Damascus, going to kill more people who were confessing this false Messiah, and he is struck blind and has a vision. He hears Christ speak to him. Christ says, "Saul, why do you persecute me?" That causes Saul of Tarsus to reconsider a lot of the assumptions that he'd been living by. He says to the voice, "Well, what do you want me to do?" The voice says, "Go into Damascus and you will find the man who will tell you what to do."

Saul goes into Damascus and repents of the idea that Christ is not the Messiah. And supposedly he spends three years in Arabia before he goes back to Jerusalem, but for our purposes, now he's Paul and now he feels like he knows where to begin. He doesn't have to be killing anybody. If we're lucky, we feel at some point that maybe this is the bridge to the world, this work. Maybe this is a way I can stand.

He goes back up to Jerusalem and says, "Men, I got it. I got the good news." He goes to James, who is Christ's brother, and to Simon, who is known as Peter. They look at him, the guy who killed one of their own, and they say, "Um, good, good. Why don't you . . . work elsewhere? Do your work elsewhere."

A guy who wants to be of the fellowship, quite literally. So humiliated, the one thing you want is to get out of the situation without having to acknowledge that you've been humiliated, so he agrees.

"You want me to go, you want me to go work. My assignment is to go work over there."

"Yeah, that's your assignment. Get away from us. Your assignment is to get away from us."

"Good, okay. So I'll work over there under your instructions."

And that's what Paul does. He goes all over the Mediterranean.

First he tries to make friends among his own, he goes to the synagogue and he says, "Christ is available to us not through the law but through faith, through the miracle. All we need to do is confess Christ crucified and resurrected. We don't have to be observant, we don't have to do the Sabbath, we don't have to be circumcised."

They beat his balls off. Every place he goes, they say, "What do you mean we don't have to do this and we don't have to do that? That's what we do." He says, "You don't have to do that. Believe me, I had a vision—this is the way it is." And so they'd beat his balls off some more.

Then, every place he went, after he gets his balls beaten off in the synagogues, he goes out among strangers and preaches Christ crucified and Christ risen. In his mind, what he would say is, "Christ told me this was not merely for the Jews but for the Gentile as well." A lot of the Gentiles aren't circumcised, so that's big. They say, "He died for me, he rose, and I don't have to be circumcised? That's it. I'm in."

Now he's getting a lot of converts and he's calling them Jews. The Jews from the synagogues notice. "What's this? They're not circumcised and they're calling themselves Jews. They're not Jews."

"It's Paul."

"I thought we threw him out."

"Well, now he's out of the synagogue, he's telling the uncircumcised they can be one of us."

"Let's beat his balls off." They go and they beat him again.

He leaves whatever community he's in and he goes to the next one. But now he begins to write back to the community that he had to flee. Every place that he's driven out of, he writes back to the fellowship, and those are the Epistles.

Paul goes back to Jerusalem after he collects tithes in all these places and he tries to get the boys to accept him one more time. He comes back, he says, "I've converted thousands of people and they have given the tithe to the holy church, the big synagogue, the big temple."

Peter and James say, "You're back and that's great. Thank you for the money." Then they turn to their guard. "Arrest this man." And they arrest him. Paul claims because he was born in a Roman colony, as a Roman citizen he has the right to be tried before Caesar. And that's how he saves his life. But consider for a moment what that was like for him to have his works rejected like that. When he leaves again, he says, "All right, so you want me in Rome. You want me working in Rome?"

"Yeah, work in Rome." And he does, and that's where he dies.

He ached to be part of something and committed murder in order to be part of it. And then somehow it was given to him to understand that that action would not, could not, make him part of a fellowship, and he repented. He had a vision that another man died for his sins so that he was washed clean. And it was in going out and sharing that message that he found real fellowship, even though he kept being told to shut the fuck up, or go away.

So a few years after Father Kieser told me to, I finally read all this about Paul, and I decide two things: "I need to teach another writing class," and "I'm gonna make a show about this guy."

* * *

The class was called The Writer's Spirit. In many ways it was about ideas I had used in my teaching for a long time, turning problems of spirit into problems of technique, but I knew I was going to integrate Paul in the course in a big way. Paul's a writer, arguably the most commercially successful writer that ever lived, and I wanted to talk about him as a writer and think about what we as writers could learn from him. I rented the auditorium at the Writers Guild Theater for five Tuesdays in a row. The first class was scheduled for September eleventh. This was 2001.

It was early in L.A. when it all started, but I was up. I felt a kind of weight of despondency descend on me, which was an appropriate response to what was happening that day, but that would alternate with a kind of manic activity and resolve. Some of those same feelings that World War II was the lead-up to my birth. I tell Rita we're keeping the kids home from school, because in my head, given they go to a fancy school with the children of some important people, that's a legitimate possible target. I have to cancel that night's lecture too, of course. I call my friend Jeff Berg, who ran ICM and happened to be Colin Powell's book agent. I ask him to come over to the house, that it's very important. I'm asking him to help me reach out to various government officials. I have some good ideas and I want to see them implemented. I am prepared to back it up with some money, the assumption being they are all bribable. Jeff is kind enough to hear all of my ideas and also kind enough to not call anyone. He and Rita only catch each other's eyes a few times. My kids, all kept home from school, wander in and out of the kitchen to get some food and see if I'm still going. So that's what I take medication for.

Now it's a week later, the eighteenth, and it's the night of the rescheduled first lecture and I'm trying to figure out what to say. I know we're going to have to talk about how we felt watching what happened. We had all received a series of images over the course of that week. As humans, we understand what those images signified. When a plane goes into a building, we understand at some level that people are dying horribly, even though we're not seeing that exactly. But the parts of our cerebellum that understand that fact are connected with other parts of our cerebrum that are typically moved to action by that perception. The analogy is you're sitting on a bus and you see a stranger get up and slap a woman. You have a natural impulse to respond. Then a whole series of absolutely legitimate considerations may intervene that keep you from responding. Maybe the guy's got a knife, maybe you're hurt, maybe you're of a particular age. But invariably, in the aftermath of failing to take action, a person becomes despondent, begins to feel useless, less than a whole person. We had all received those images of the terrible loss of life, and to the extent that we'd been unable to respond in the instinctual human fashion that we've evolved over whatever hundreds of thousands of years, we become sad. We become despondent. We feel ineffectual.

I want us all to name those feelings, because that's what writers feel when we're not writing. Inadequate, untalented, incompetent, unworthy.

I'm talking all of this through with the class, and I've already showed them I brought my Bible with me, and about thirty minutes in I say, "You know what might be useful, maybe I could ask one or two or four of you to share the parts of this past week, watching what went on on television or as you experienced it personally, that you found uplifting."

One woman gets up to a microphone and I ask her name and she says her name's Susan. We had these classes recorded, this was all transcribed. I interrupt her, "You know what would be a good thing too? Each of you should whisper your name to the person on either side of you." So everyone does that. Then Susan says, "Hearing of the phone calls that people made, making a last communication, in particular, the phone call of, I don't remember his name, on Flight 93, when he was calling his wife and we sort of got a communication through her of their decision that they were going to take some sort of action, that they knew that they were going to die and they were going to do whatever they could."

A guy named Mark says, "I don't know if this is uplifting but it was in Sunday's paper. They had a whole big article about people escaping from the building, one of the towers. There was one guy, one of the nicest guys in the building—it was sort of a building where a lot of backstabbing goes on and this sort of thing. This guy, who was a father of two, well liked, he went down, and he caught up with a guy who was going, a very fat guy, tremendously obese, who had started on like the seventieth floor, and he'd gone to the fiftieth floor and he couldn't go anymore, and he stopped with this guy and he and other people said, 'You've got to keep going.' And the fat guy said, 'I just can't, I can't go on anymore.' And this guy said, 'Well I'm not leaving.' I don't know if it was uplifting, or what it was. I tried to see myself in that situation. I don't know if I would or not."

Another woman mentions the firefighter parade. Someone

talks about the Linda Ellerbee special, kids saying we shouldn't bomb anyone in response because making other people hurt wouldn't help. One guy talks about the Braves game, hearing people sing "Take Me Out to the Ball Game."

Then I ask, what do all those moments have in common? They begin with an individual and culminate in the individual finding the deepest meaning of his individuality in a going-out to something outside himself or herself. One of the corollaries of that explains the impulse to get up and give blood, the impulse to send groceries, the impulse to go down and serve coffee.

Every person has in their heart the capacity, when encouraged by a benign organizing presence, to identify the deepest truths of the human story. Four people got up in a room of hundreds and did it for nothing other than being given the chance.

The main writing exercise I like to give students is an attempt to make it easier to do that, easier to give yourself that chance. Here it is:

For the next five days, find a time each day, preferably the same time, and sit down and write not less than twenty minutes and not more than fifty minutes. Five-zero. Don't think about it, don't set it up on the computer, don't think about what you're going to write before you do it. No exceptions. This means you.

Two voices, one and two. No names. No description. No description. That means no description. Voice one and voice two. The setting—don't say what the setting is. No description. Write for not less than twenty minutes with those two voices. Just follow, just hear what they say. Not more than fifty minutes. Put it in an envelope, seal the envelope, and shut up. Don't talk about it. Don't think about what it means. Don't think about who they are.

The next day, preferably at the same time, sit down and do it again. They may be the same voices, they may be different voices, don't worry about it. Whatever comes out is fine. Don't think about it. Just do it.

In the course of these exercises, the true categories of your imagination emerge, and they are absolutely different from what you think they are. What the exercises do is build certain neural pathways and shut down certain other neural pathways. It's a physiological and a behavioral sequence that creates neurological changes. It is a way of habituating yourself in a different fashion, and you can't fool around with it.

It's like when you're learning how to drive. You get in the car and you're filled with fear and God forbid it's your mother or your father teaching you how to drive, because then maybe even you're afraid of getting hit. But, even if it's a teacher, the thing you might feel is, "I'm the one who can't do it. I'm never going to learn because it's too much, it's too many things, every decision is individual."

If you had to drive that way it would be a misery. But what you find is that if you repeat the behaviors over a not-significant period of time, say three weeks, and you take the lessons, and then you sit and talk with a friend, what you will probably confide is, "I was always able to drive. I dunno, I was born that way. I mean I just know how to drive." That's because you have set up a series of neural connections so that one behavior instinctually generates the impulse to do the next behavior.

Our ideas about what we are or can do or want, those can change.

The class went on like that for five weeks, plus me reading

the Bible a lot. I suppose I was at a stage in my sobriety where I was more hospitable to that. A *Los Angeles Times* article about that class called it "the church of Milch." But there are those who knew me before I became a religious fanatic. I can watch the tapes of that class now and I seem on the verge of something, and maybe even happy.

* * *

After that I was ready to get this Paul show together. I wanted the show to be at the end of Paul's life, after the rejection, the conversion, the traveling and the Epistles, when he got to Rome. Nero was emperor when Paul got there, and things were pretty fucked, which will happen when a whole society is structured around the whims of a psychopath. I read Suetonius, I read Tacitus, Livy. There was so much to read. There were two sets of cops in Rome then, the Praetorian Guard and the Urban Cohort. The Praetorian Guard were basically the palace cops, so that was very straightforward, you just do whatever it is Nero wants. Cut out someone's tongue and tie it around their neck? Absolutely, no problem. Do the hands too. But the Urban Cohort, they were the city cops, so it's still ultimately Nero's rules but also they're dealing with people in the streets, fighting over plumbing or who a slave belongs to and other beefs that don't necessarily have anything to do with Nero. But you've also got the Senate, the wealthier families, a lot of competing considerations. How do you figure out what the rules are in a place like that? You know they only apply insofar as they don't piss off the emperor, but also you don't want people killing each other in the street (except the emperor, for him it's fine). The show was about the head of the Urban Cohort, and I imagined he was also a father, and he just wanted to figure out a way to protect his family in what could otherwise be a sort of precarious existence. And so when Paul gets to Rome and starts preaching a new faith that says that the way one should live in fact has nothing to do with what the madman in the palace wants at any given moment, the way to live is to embrace Christ's love, and all you have to believe in is the symbol of Christ's suffering, the cross, that's going to louse things up for the emperor, and a whole bunch of other people. So the city cops are told to arrest Paul, and that was going to be the first episode. And then, one of the main cop's sons was going to become a follower of Paul, which would have put his dad in an especially tough spot once Nero started calling for Paul's followers to be burned alive. And while Paul is in Rome waiting for trial, Nero starts the Great Fire, blames it on the Christians (even though he is actually just trying to make room for the new estate he wants to build), but still people keep converting, and the city starts to change, even as Nero keeps getting wackier to try to keep things how they were, until he knows it's beyond him. What interested me in that story was the extent to which adherence to the symbol of a thing, the cross, galvanized energy, and in fact compounded the availability of energy, and how over time that truly changed Rome.

So I went into HBO and pitched this series and it's an hour-long pitch and I finish and they say, "That's the best pitch we ever heard. The only thing is, we're already doing a show about Rome." It's like the story about the obnoxious Jewish couple—they want to give their kid a bar mitzvah where no one else has had a bar mitzvah, so they decide they're going to have a bar mitzvah in Kenya. And they hire the rabbi, they hire all the elephants to take them into the woods, and there's this long line of elephants and finally the line of elephants comes to a stop and the father of the lucky boy asks the guy, "What's the problem? What's the holdup?" And the guide says, "We got to wait, there's another bar mitzvah ahead of us."

It's a credit to Chris Albrecht and Carolyn Strauss, who were the HBO executives I was pitching, that instead of just having me escorted out of the room, they asked, "Can you give us the same story somewhere else?" I understood the story I wanted to tell, and it wasn't necessarily about the specific incidents in Rome, though I had to learn all those incidents before I went in and pitched it. What I had been interested in was how Paul's coming to proselytize had offered a different symbol around which people could organize. The symbol had been the emperor and Paul was now offering the cross. So when they said, "Well, we're already doing a show about Rome," I said, "Okay, I know another symbol that man organized around, which is gold." I could set the show somewhere gold had just been discovered. The agreement to act as if gold had a particular value, and organize behavior around that collective agreement, was really the same story. Gold is a lie agreed upon. There is no intrinsic value in gold. It's only the energy that it liberates in the people who believe in it. We have to find the lie to agree upon that allows us to live together so that we can address this larger concern. There's a fancy term called metempsychosis, which is the transmigration of spirits, reincarnation. Being able to see the same spirit moving in different places, different settings, different people and stories, that's one of the blessings of art. I believe that comes in part from prayer and an open heart to the possibilities of the day, and if the possibilities of that day include someone saying, "There's a bar mitzvah ahead of you," you may be willing to say, "Sure, we'll make it a Western. Let me go figure it out and I'll be back in a few months."

* * *

Rita started stacking books again. I ended up reading for about six months. I like research. It probably reminds me of when I was working with my teachers. I'd spend days in the stacks at Sterling, or in the reading rooms at Beinecke (that's where I found some love letters Edith Wharton had written that no one had ever seen before when I was working with Dick Lewis on his Wharton book). Discovering histories, layering up impressions, building one upon the other. It's fun.

I knew gold would work as an initial organizing principle, releasing people's energy the same as the cross, and then I knew I wanted a place that was out on a frontier, not yet incorporated into the United States. States were getting incorporated fast in the mid-1800s, especially in the far west, then there's a pretty big gap between Nebraska in 1867 and Colorado in 1876, and then no more new states until 1889, when the Dakotas, Montana, and Washington were all incorporated in the span of two weeks. I liked the idea of telling a story set after the Industrial Revolution, when everyone senses that things are changing fast. As I did my research, I got very interested in a settlement in the Black Hills of the Dakota Territory. Custer had been there in 1874 in the Battle of Little Big Horn and started saying there was gold then, but the real find came in 1876, and in about fifteen days the camp went from fifty to five thousand people. It ended up being the largest gold strike in the country, and what became the Homestake Mine would be the start of the Hearst family fortune. I said to Rita, "Get any book you can find about a town called Deadwood."

Dutton's Books was still open then on San Vicente Boulevard, and she'd go there and get what they had and ask them to order even more. There was a book called *Pioneer Days in the Black Hills: Accurate History and Facts Related by One of the Early Day Pioneers*. This guy named John McClintock arrived in Deadwood in April 1876. A woman named Estelline Bennett arrived as a little girl in 1877, her dad was a judge and supposed to help reform the place. There weren't too many kids in the town when they first got there. She wrote a book called *Old Deadwood Days*. There were a number of books by a historian named Watson Parker.

The other thing that interested me in particular about Deadwood was that it was a criminal enterprise, and it acknowledged itself as a criminal enterprise. There was no law in Deadwood because it was an illegal settlement. It was on land that had been stolen from the Native Americans, and not just in the way the whole country was stolen, although that too, but this land had explicitly been given to the Sioux in the Fort Laramie Treaty. There was a concern by the thieves, meaning the white prospectors, that if they passed any laws, they would be perceived as setting up their own government, and that would get their land taken away. They wanted to be annexed to the United States, they wanted their claims verified by the United States, but they knew they couldn't get ahead of themselves with laws, so they agreed that there would be no law whatsoever.

That meant booze, prostitution, opium, theft—all fair game. During the summer of 1876 there was a murder a day in the town. On any day, there was a not insignificant chance for any person there that they'd get killed. And if they did get killed, the body would more likely be burned or fed to pigs than buried so that there would be no evidence, so that there could be no trial, so that nobody could say that they had set up a government. Even famous people. When Wild Bill Hickok was killed they acquitted the guy who killed him. Twice. Because if they recognized even one kind of law then someone would have had the right to say you just stole all this from the Sioux.

Now who is drawn to a place like that? A lot of people who for one reason or another are willing to take the risk that they might die, or maybe even a little bit want to (or a lot, as it seemed to me was the case for Wild Bill as I read about him). Once that's who's coming to a place, it just gets crazier.

And yet. When the plague came, they set up tents and Jane Cannary helped the local doctor treat the sick people (that's how she got her nickname—Calamity Jane). A minister named Henry Weston Smith felt called to come to the town and preach. A guy named A. W. Merrick got to town and set up a newspaper, the *Black Hills Pioneer* (which is still independent and running today). A pair of friends who'd met in Montana came to town to open a hardware store together and eventually wound up becoming sheriff and mayor. They bought the lot for their store from Al Swearengen, the pimp who ran the Gem Saloon, who never once kneeled in the creeks but made about five grand a day off the men who did.

Reading about this town, how society forms, how America came to be, how people make a community whether they intend to or not, it was all there.

The other thing that started to feel good was that thinking about that period, in America, made me feel close to my teachers, and to the writers we had read and talked so much about. Melville and Hawthorne and Twain and the James brothers, Stephen Crane and Sarah Orne Jewett, Wharton and Cather, everything I had read, everything I knew about them was coming back into play.

So I went back to Carolyn and Chris and pitched them *Deadwood* and they bought it. One wrinkle was that I was still under contract at Paramount when we sold the show. In the subsequent negotiation, since it was clear I wasn't gonna stay at Paramount once my deal was up, in order to release me and the show to HBO, Paramount got the rights to the international sales of *Deadwood*. That would end up being of some import later on but was absolutely in the category of things I didn't give a fuck about or really pay attention to at the time. I was just excited to get to work.

That's how the show about Christianity in ancient Rome became a show about gold in the American West. I didn't teach the class I thought I was going to teach or make the show I thought I was going to make. If you want to hear God laugh, tell Him your plans.

6.

Owl at Dawn

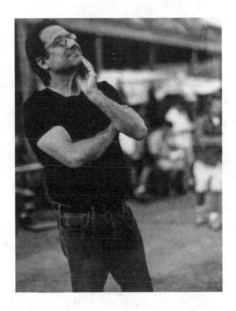

It seemed so obvious to me that the West I had encountered in my research had nothing to do with the Westerns I had experienced as a kid—*Hopalong Cassidy, The Cisco Kid*—which weren't even good on their own terms. They didn't interest me particularly even then. And going back and watching some classic Westerns, those too had very little to do with the West that I was studying (though they told some good stories). Then I did some research to figure out how *that* had happened, how the Westerns of the thirties, forties, and fifties had developed, and what I discovered was that it had everything to do with what Hollywood was about at that time, and nothing to do with what the West was about.

There had been a period of five or ten years in the late teens and early twenties where films had gotten a little racy. The dream factory was operated exclusively by immigrant Jews, but then some of the other popular thinkers of the twenties were guys like Charles Lindbergh and Henry Ford, who were saying, "We've got to do something, the moneylenders are taking over," and worse than that. The Goldwyns and Lanskys and Mayers and Zanucks wanted to stay behind the scenes and keep making their movies and their money, and in order to keep doing that they wanted to send a message that they weren't going to rock the boat any more in terms of the stories they were telling. They got together and hired a front Gentile named Hays, who instituted what was called the Hays Production Code that proclaimed, "Obscenity [. . .] in spoken word, gesture, episode, plot, is against divine and human law, and hence altogether outside the range of subject matter or treatment." That was the guys in Hollywood saying, let us run the show, and you will get 150 features a year that glorify innocence and an absence of conflict. And those rules governed all of television and film from 1934 to 1968.

But there's no rule that can stop art, though there are plenty that will change it. If you're an artist, when you're confronted with those kinds of strictures, you can refuse to participate or you can try and find a way to internalize them such that it doesn't distort the story you're trying to tell. And so some of the great storytellers in films of the thirties and forties extrapolated a character who was very laconic. Not only didn't use swear words, this character just didn't talk much at all. His stoicism invoked a whole set of values. There is a way to make a character like that credible, and that's part of what I saw in the historical Bullock and would explore in that character. But that's just one way to be, and I believed that would be a pretty rare, if important, type of person, very much the exception rather than the rule, and that what made him that way would be as dark and complicated, obscene let's say, as anyone else.

I had done my research. I had also asked one of my horse trainers, Darrell Vienna, if he knew any cowboys I should meet. He introduced me to a guy named Gary Leffew, who has his own bull riding school in Central California and is in the Bull Riding Hall of Fame, that's a real thing.

Darrell also helped me oversee the sale of the ten Thoroughbred I owned in August of 2002, which is called a dispersal. I wanted to be free of that addiction too. I knew it was the right thing to do because it put me in a slippery place. I didn't want to be embarrassed by fucking up. But I mourned that loss, even more than the other things I'd given up, because it was so much associated with my dad. There was the slow process of discovering, of living into, the healing of the soul. I sold almost all my horses then, ended up keeping a minority stake in a couple because of how the sales shook out, but I wasn't going to the track, which was big. I didn't want to go between work and the track. I just wanted to work.

So Darrell and I visited Gary's bull riding school, and I started spending some time with Gary. We decided he'd get together a group of rodeo cowboys and we'd all take a short trip to Deadwood, to the town. They've turned it into a kind of tourist destination but a lot of the places are still there and there was a library and historical society I wanted to visit and I figured who better to go to the town with than some cowboys. First I flew them all to Los Angeles, put them up for a night or two here, then I got us a plane to Deadwood. Gary got a wild crew, eight or nine guys, all different kinds. I didn't drink but they sure did. A few of them had maybe killed people, a few of them sang. Some loved their animals. They all best knew how to live the eight or so seconds they were riding a bull, and all the rest of the time they were just trying to figure out what the fuck to do with themselves. Seeing that so crystallized in them, that was probably the greatest gift they gave me.

Every day, before I start to write, I pray, and I ask to be willing, and then I see what happens. "I offer myself to Thee to build with me and do with me as Thou wilt. Relieve me of the bondage of self, that I may better do Thy will." People who've been in recovery might recognize that as the third-step prayer, and that's the one I say every day. It's my asking to have the perspective of self lifted and to give myself to the situation and the characters. I find that I function most effectively when I sort of disembody myself. I lie there on the floor and I talk and the words come up on the screen and then I fix the words, but I never actually lay my hands on anything, a computer or a typewriter, none of that.

It was time to listen, to find the characters up and walking and hear who they were and what they had to say. In everything I read about the West, and gold camps in particular, one thing about which there was uniform agreement was the language that was used in these communities. The extremity of the language was, in its own way, one of the few alternatives to law. The same way that an ape may beat his chest to signify his willingness to do something that, if he had to do it every time he signified his willingness, he'd be in fights all the time, the obscenity was one alternative for people in the camps, and it was a crucial alternative for me to portray in the absence of these other ordering mechanisms. If you went out to an environment like this it wasn't because you were doing great in Wilkes-Barre, Pennsylvania. There were some personality attributes, maybe there was a warrant or two out. Because there were no laws, any question potentially had lethal implications. If I say, "Where are you from?" you're usually gonna say where you're from. In Deadwood, if you say, "Where are you from?," the response was, "What the fuck is that to you?" Immediately it becomes a potentially mortal situation. It was a way of announcing, "Don't come in here with any weak shit." But the obscenity is not indiscriminate. It's calibrated according to the given personality and the given environment. The obscenity is meant to do a lot of different things.

The language, it seemed to me, had to serve two functions. The first was to beat down the viewers' preexisting expectation that any law would be obeyed, sentences so soaked with obscenity as to bleach out the expectation that civility could be expected to govern in any given scene. To ask the viewer to live in that emotional environment with the characters, that was the first part of it. The second part was that I wanted to show how words generated meaning not because of any intrinsic quality but because of the context of emotional association in which they were expressed. The meaning would come from the community we build around and through the words. As the series unfolds, I wanted to show language complicating itself as one of the alternatives to statute, that people come to govern their own behavior as much through language as through law.

I was also interested in the patterns of speech and the distinction between people who had what was called book learning and people who didn't. The people who had book learning tended to speak in an almost Elizabethan way. This was Victorian times. For those who had book learning, it was the Bible, Shakespeare, Dickens, Victorian literature, plus adventure stories, but that access wasn't strictly tied to class. There's a story about Kit Carson riding seven days to get his new collection of

Sir Walter Scott. It seemed to me that the people in that environment who had recourse to books were highly, highly motivated. It was an alternative state of being for them, which stood in contrast to the way they were living. And so I found it credible that people who had recourse to that sort of rhetoric would go for the gusto. Trying to get those rhythms right was a challenge, but it was one I very much enjoyed. Most of the show is written in iambic pentameter. I believe one way God says, "I too have a hand here" is in the rhythms and metrics of speech, that the metrics of speech are important and representative of our fellowship even in those of us who feel, mistakenly, that we are separate from each other as individuals. When a character in Deadwood, or anyone, talks in certain locutions, unbeknownst to themselves, they honor a divine presence.

* * *

When I taught that class, after three weeks of the two-voice exercises, I asked everyone to introduce a third voice. It could be a new character, it could be a narrator, but instead of just two voices, they had to bring someone new on the scene. That fucked everyone up. The fourth Tuesday we met, every person I asked, it was the same story: "The exercises were going so great, I felt good, then I tried to do the third voice, and I couldn't figure it out. I got so depressed." Whether it's a narrator or a third voice, our uneasiness in relation to that is the inevitable consequence of our ambivalence about form, about the structuring forces in the world—every writer will have to live into that eventually. The feeling outside things, that's the burden of our identity; it's also its source. We are people who feel ambivalent enough about the world that we are compelled to imagine other worlds. Feeling that kind of ambivalence is uncomfortable. It can be an excuse not to practice our art, if we want it to be. Or we can accept our discomfort—that's just the way it is, and it's also the source of all beauty. Without form, we simply have a series of chaotic significations; that's no way to live.

When I was writing *Deadwood*, my formal voice changed. I was writing more scene description than I'd ever written before. Not parenthetical adjectives about a line reading (I still hated those) but things like this on Swearengen:

> He drinks, in his element, widening his horizons to consider other impositions by Fate on the smooth enactment of his will—

The reason that happened then I think is that I accepted that the formal voice is God's voice. No matter how you distort it or reverb it, it's still God's voice. Once you accept that, when you're writing, the question becomes, what would be necessary to God, if the narrator has to be true to the narrator's nature and the characters have to be true to their natures? If we were to say that God as a narrator wants to place the characters in a situation most congenial to their discovery of their deepest nature—which is that their sense of themselves as separate is predicated on an utter misapprehension, and they are all one thing—how would you go about telling that story?

That book by John McClintock, *Pioneer Days in the Black Hills*, there was so much in it. The day a prostitute named Tricksie shot a guy in the head and he was still talking after. I didn't like that spelling but I liked that story. Bullock and Hickok arrived in the camp within three days of each other, that's one where I took a liberty and made it the same day. There was a Metz family murdered by road agents, but they didn't have a child, let alone three. Cleanth Brooks taught me there are different kinds of truths, and that while the truths of reportage or history depend upon a correspondence to an externally verifiable reality, the truths of storytelling are the truths of an internal emotional coherence. Melville called it the very truth. I felt as long as I was telling the very truth, I was okay.

I knew I wanted Swearengen to be as central as Bullock, that in his own way he was important to the camp growing too. Having a bar, and taking money in payment for liquor or women, creates a society, and it's a mistake to identify that type of society as different from, say, a family, if people devote their energies to it and find their relaxation there. What I thought I was going to show through Swearengen was that growing a government can be a great way to run the long con, or keep control of the money, and that's one way you get what we think of as civilization. I wanted Ed O'Neill to play Swearengen, that's who I first wrote it for, but HBO wouldn't go. They wouldn't cast him because it ain't television. It's HBO. Then we cast Powers Boothe, but Powers got sick for the first time right before we were supposed to shoot the pilot. I told him I'd write a different part for him to play when he got well, but we had to go ahead and shoot. Ian McShane came in to read for the part and physically he was so different from what I had imagined, arguably wrong for the part as I had originally conceived of it, but he came in and read and showed me who Swearengen was. When that happens, you have to be humble enough to say, "Forget how I pictured it. This is the guy." What Swearengen became, how his language developed, the soliloquies, that was all because Ian could do it. He'd get pages hot from the printer and he enjoyed it because he knew how good he was. He's an athlete.

All the characters, I really came to know them like that, as we found our actors. We were shooting the pilot in October of 2002. Junie Lowry-Johnson and Libby Goldstein were our casting directors; they're just very good. Junie had done the casting on *NYPD Blue* too. We had so much time together that we could talk a little about what I was thinking for a character and they just got it, or they would surprise me and show me someone who was totally different than what I was thinking, and better. A lot of the actors on *Deadwood* had done an episode or two with us. They say when people show you who they are, believe them. That's true enough, but don't stop looking either, because there's more to see.

Some actors came in to audition in costume, and that works if you're a good actor. There was a quite prominent actor who auditioned in full Wild Bill Hickok regalia, and I hated him with a mortal passion (I can't remember who now, I wouldn't say even if I did). But then Robin Weigert came in full Jane drag, and she was just great. There are those moments when you know right then in the room, the search is done. Somehow Robin and I were on the same flight to New York the next day, and I asked the flight attendants if I could move to sit next to her, and we talked the whole flight, and that's when I really learned who Calamity Jane would be. There was no corner of Jane that Robin was scared to put a light to. We hadn't cast Wild Bill yet and we talked together about who Bill might be, what different Bills might mean to Jane. I carried her costume bag through the airport when we got off. When an actor is ready like that, you just want them to know you're ready to do whatever you can to help them on their way.

We found our Bill in Keith Carradine, our Bullock in Tim Olyphant. I remember watching Tim in *Go*, a totally different kind of part, but you had to have a wildness underneath in Bullock that he was just barely keeping at bay. Tim had been a swimmer in college. You could watch him move through the town, breaking through water, muscles working in his back. Molly Parker, who would play Alma, had been a ballerina starting when she was three. I always thought Alma would become a writer, someone like Willa Cather, and that was something Molly and I talked about from the very start, that that was where she was headed, that part of why she used opium was that ambivalence about her reality. Trixie was supposed to die early in the show but Paula Malcomson made me see that she couldn't. Paula so immediately occupied the character that even before we finished the pilot I was just running around trying to catch up. It would have been an act of impiety not to listen. Geri Jewell I had seen in line at the pharmacy. I told her I was a big fan, but I hadn't seen her in much since *The Facts of Life*. She was recovering from spinal surgery, picking up her medication. I asked if she would be in the show I was working on. She said, "This is a pharmacy, right?" She was the first person cast. We met at my office at Paramount and talked about the time period and what it would be like to be disabled then and I asked her to write what she thought her character would be like. She sent me twenty pages and she was a great writer. I told her I liked ninety-nine percent of it but I didn't like the name. Geri wanted her to be called Crazy Kate. I said, "No. Her name is going to be Jewel."

Walter Hill came on to direct the pilot. He had directed a great film called *The Warriors* and had a real knowledge of and respect for the whole history of the Western, had even directed a movie called *Wild Bill*, and that respect would allow us to play with it. Janie Bryant had done the costumes on *Big Apple*, and she joined up again. Walter brought on a production designer named Maria Caso, and beyond directing the pilot, bringing Maria on was his huge and lasting contribution to the show.

Maria's work, along with that of our art director, James Murakami, was just sensational.

We shot at Melody Ranch in Santa Clarita. They had made *The Lone Ranger* and *Gunsmoke* there, then for about forty years Gene Autry kept it as a ranch for his horse. It's a twenty-two-acre lot with offices and three soundstages, everything you need to never leave. When the sun was out it could be a hundred degrees and when the sun was down it was freezing. Maria and James built a town, they built a world. The Grand Central Hotel, you walked in from the street and you were in the lobby. The front desk was to your right and the dining room to your left and you walked up the stairs and there was Alma's suite. The Gem was across the street, with Al's balcony, looking out at the whole town. The inside of the Gem was on a soundstage, but you walked into that door from the Gem on the street, and it was two stories, you could walk up the stairs and through the hall and into Al's room. Even for the pilot, the main thoroughfare was the length of a couple football fields, and Chinatown Alley was a backstreet, and Doc's cabin was around the bend. There were horses there every day, tents, mud. I could walk through the street and get ideas for new scenes, just reading the hand-painted signs. It was all so alive. Shooting that pilot, all you could think was, "Gee, I hope we get to keep doing this."

HBO gave us a series order at the start of 2003. That February I was given the Eustace D. Theodore Fellowship at Yale. Eustace had been the dean of Calhoun College when I was teaching and he would see me climbing into my office through the window because I had locked myself out. The theme of the fellowship was The Curious Use of a Yale Education, so I was to give one talk on that and another, at the law school I had been kicked out of, on the future of the television drama. They gave Rita and me a suite in the college. She didn't enjoy that much because a visiting poet had tried to assault her in that same room when she was an undergraduate, though she didn't explain that to me until after the weekend. We did a screening of a rough cut of the pilot at the Whitney Humanities Center. The last screening I had there was a short film called *Pilgrims* in 1973 that I wrote and acted in. It's set at a truck stop, just two truckers talking, the one I played vacillating between uppers and downers. The other trucker is strange and annoying but he just keeps talking and my character just keeps talking back, doesn't know why, can't help himself, is sort of shocked the whole time that the conversation continues. Mr. Warren had attended that screening, and it just meant so much to me. I don't think I even told my parents about it. I wasn't that young then, twenty-eight already, but still so unformed, didn't know if I'd ever get it together. Then I was back there at fifty-eight, and in a certain way I think it was the first time I felt like I had made good. My eldest was a freshman then, and she brought all her new friends to my talks. We had dinner with Mr. Theodore. The work I was showing then, the pilot, the sound wasn't finished, and we would end up reshooting the opening scene, but it felt worthy of Mr. Warren watching. He wasn't there but it felt worthy.

* * *

We started shooting again that summer. In the time between, I had been editing the pilot, thinking about the stories for the season, thinking about the characters, but I'd only written about two more scripts. And once we were shooting again, there was just so much the actors were bringing to it, and we'd figure out new things together, get new ideas, change it. I'll tell you when my understanding of some of the characters really started to shift.

We were shooting the second episode. I knew that Swearengen was supposed to kill this little girl, the little Norwegian girl whose family had been murdered by road agents who tried to make it look like the Sioux had done it. I couldn't write it. She's in Doc's cabin, still fighting for her life. Jane is guarding her. I finally said to Ian McShane, "Go in there, think you're gonna kill her, and have it turn out that you can't." That scene became something else entirely. It became about Swearengen seeing that the little girl was alive and about Jane becoming afraid of Swearengen, and hating herself for being afraid, because it made her feel like when she was a little girl and had to prostitute herself to survive (which she did, and somehow we got Doris Day). And changing that scene meant the next scene had to change. It was Al walking back from Doc's cabin and Doc—Brad Dourif— walking toward it and nothing was written but I told Brad and Ian, just walk toward each other. I told Brad, "As you're walking, you're thinking, if she's dead, it's because I've failed, it's because of everything wrong with me, you think you might be walking toward the verdict on your whole life, but you're also thinking at least now I'll know, and then you start to think, 'Well, there's also the chance she's okay.'" So they start walking toward each other, and the lines start to come, I called them out to them:

COCHRAN

Did you hurt her?

SWEARENGEN

No. No, Doc. But she's better than you thought. Her eyes are open.

Then it was gonna be that Swearengen has Dan kill the little girl. But it happened again. I couldn't write it that way. The scene became about Doc standing firm, saying Dan would have to kill him too, and Dan, with tears in his eyes, so relieved because he didn't want to do it. They find Jane and Charlie in the thoroughfare and have them take the little girl. By the time they are back at the Gem to tell Al, he's dealt with the problem another way, killing the last living road agent instead. That sequence, it liberated my perception of the characters—the show would be about isolated constructive gestures, and how out of those isolated constructive gestures, a little girl is saved, and the society begins to build itself. The episode ends with Jane and Charlie singing to the girl in a round,

> *Row row row your boat*
> *Gently down the stream*
> *Merrily merrily merrily*
> *Life is but a dream.*

If you're sticking with your work, you discover truths about it that aren't present when you begin, and that's the real fun. Symbols, signifiers, they generate their meaning out of the submission of energy from the believer. They're fluid rather than stable. They mean different things at different times. The same nugget of gold can be a source of wealth or it can be a source of destruction. The symbolism as it strengthens and stabilizes generates more and more complicated social institutions.

The poet Coleridge attempted to distinguish between fanciful and imaginative associations. If I hear Del Shannon's "Runaway" and I think of the first time I had sex, that's a fanciful association because it so happened that record was playing when I first had sex. There is nothing inherent in the experience of listening to Del Shannon's "Runaway" that would make *you* think of the first time *I* had sex. If we see a bird fly and we both think of freedom, that's because there is something inherent in the bird's flying, and that's an imaginative association an artist can tap into. A child, children, they generate in or offer to us all sorts of imaginative associations. Innocence, vulnerability, a future, need, accountability, hope. The camp's care for Sofia, over time, is as much in who stays away as in who steps in to care. When Swearengen and Dan forbear, they give her a chance. There are people who care for her, then take their leave. Jane, Doc, Charlie, Trixie, Joanie. They give her what they can when they can. And there is Alma, who gives up things she might want in order to take on Sofia's care, and Ellsworth, who joins up to help her. That's how a child learns to trust the world—the world earns their trust. That doesn't mean nothing bad happens.

My kids were older when I was working on *Deadwood*, teens, college. I was getting a premium of Rita's attention in a way I hadn't since before we had kids. I'll admit I liked that. The kids' attention too, because they were older, they could help, they could participate. Elizabeth interned with Maria Caso in the art department in the summer, later Ben would too. They would all come to set. Rita would bring the dogs and we'd take them to see the horses, they loved the mud. My family and dogs coming to the set, I felt happy knowing my collaborators could see that. It was important for them to see. We were talking about family constantly, and children. So many scenes, what we were really saying was, "This is a family." I could still be short-tempered or withdrawn or impatient, but I could also be present more than ever before, and they could see me love my family and our dogs.

The most fundamental difference between my children and me is that for a long time—my childhood and most of my adult life too—I wasn't able to trust the world, and my kids can. When they were kids I could see it, I knew it to be true, and it was the thing I cared about most and wanted to do whatever I could to protect. A lot of times that meant staying out of it. The first time that I watched our oldest child play in a soccer game, it was very tough for me because I wanted to fix the game. I wanted to talk to the referee. I wanted to talk to the other coach. But finally, I just had to stand back, and that's difficult, but there's an enormous release in being able to separate from the things you love. It's the beginning of peace, in a certain way. But sometimes too it meant literally staying away. Because there were other soccer games when I didn't stand back, and I got thrown out of the game, and my own kids ended up crying, and their cousins and two of their friends who were also on the team were pretty freaked out too. They were scared and embarrassed and pissed off, and when they felt that way the best thing their mother and I could do after to help them keep trusting the world was let them know they weren't wrong.

Eventually, through them, through work, through sobriety, I came to trust the world again too. When we were working on Melody Ranch I trusted it down to the ground, trusted the air, trusted the people around me every day. I wanted them to know they could trust me too, and they did, and then we were flying.

* * *

The actors told me their characters' deepest truths. They gave themselves up, and they inhabited the parts they had come to. A lot of times they might not even think they had, but they just couldn't help it. Like the rest of us, there are actors in whom fear predominates, with the exception of certain situations or moments. You try to find for that actor a situation or moment congenial to the circumvention of the fear, and then that liberates them to act in faith, in more and more different kinds of moments. "Well, I might not be able to do it, but let's give it a shot." And people are so happy when they act in faith. Even, and especially, as they overcome fear. I've seen so many actors experience the most profound kind of joy as they discover that all of the rules that they have insisted upon for so long need not necessarily apply.

Willie Sanderson, he'd beat himself up pretty good before a scene, so I made that part of the character. I remember Tim Olyphant telling me once that when he would fight as a kid, if he was winning, he'd start to cry. That's how I wrote the scene with Bullock getting tears in his eyes when he goes to beat McCall in the freezer. Wu didn't have any lines in the pilot, and I asked Keone Young to believe me that the character would be much more than what we first saw. We would write his Chinese dialogue together. I'd give him the words in English and Keone would translate them. Keone eventually came up with the idea for Wu to cut his queue, to show Swearengen he had earned Wu's trust. Dayton Callie once thought the coat Janie Bryant had picked for him was too froufrou, fought her on it, so they came to ask me what I thought. I said, "Oh, that's great." Charlie's next five scenes, I had him ask whoever he was talking to, "What do you think of this jacket? Think the tailor took it a little too far?" I got to know Dayton between *NYPD Blue* and *Deadwood*, when he was trying to help a family member who had some of the same struggles I had. The way Charlie Utter tries to help, to take care of others, the way he keeps at it whether it works or doesn't, I learned that about Charlie through Dayton.

By the third episode of the first season there usually wasn't too much of a script before we started shooting. I was writing in one trailer on the set, and the editing bay was in another trailer. We had a sense of the story and an idea of who needed to be on call each day, though sometimes that would change. All the writers were in a room. I'd lie on the floor, and the rest of the writing staff would be sitting on a couch or in chairs around me, and the monitor was facing us, and then George or Scott Willson or Taylor Toole or Zack Whedon or Nick Towne or Abby Gewanter would sit behind the desk. Some writers would just be on for an episode, but the staff, Liz Sarnoff, Regina Corrado, Jody Worth, they were almost always there. Ted Mann, who had worked with me on *NYPD Blue* many years too, was the only one who'd stay for the scene discussion but not the actual writing. It made him too crazy, which is how you know he's a halfway healthy person.

Every scene generated in that one stinking trailer fifty yards from the set, or on the set itself. All storytelling is collaborative in one way or another. Nobody writes an episode independently. Once the scene is generated, we don't let it ripen particularly, usually the scene was written either the day it's shot or the day before. No finished script before the shooting begins. If the shoot was an average of twelve days, the script was finished on the twelfth day of the shoot. The idea of being an auteur, I don't believe in that. I don't care whose name is on a script. We are organs of a larger organism which knows us although we do not know it. I regard myself as a vessel of whatever that larger organism is, its instrument, rather than as the source of the scenes. So a lot of what I do is try to get out of the way. That's the way I work on my writing. That's the way I work with the actors. That's the way I edit. It put me in the path of an enormous amount of energy.

And what about St. Paul? Where did he go? In that first season, Reverend Smith became a sort of avatar for Paul. His

sermon at Wild Bill Hickok's funeral in the fifth episode, that's
where Paul, and what I wanted the show to be about, and what
I believe about us as a species, is expressed in its purest form:

SMITH

Mr. Hickok will lie beside two brothers. One he likely
killed, the other he killed for certain, and he's been
killed now in turn. So much blood, and on the
battlefields of The Brothers' War I saw more blood
than this, and asked then after the purpose and did
not know, and don't know the purpose now, but know
now to testify that, not knowing, I believe. St. Paul
tells us, "By one Spirit are we all baptized into one
body, whether we be Jew or Gentile, bond or free,
and have all been made to drink into one Spirit. For
the body is not one member but many." He tells us,
"The eye cannot say unto the hand, I have no need of
thee; nor again the head to the feet, I have no need of
thee. Nay, much more those members of the body
which seem to be more feeble, and those members of
the body which we think of as less honorable, all are
necessary." He says that "there should be no schism
in the body, but that the members should have the
same care, one to another, and whether one member
suffer, all the members suffer with it." I believe in
God's purpose, not knowing it. I ask Him, moving in
me, to allow me to see His will. I ask Him, moving in
others, to allow them to see it.

There's good evidence that Paul was what's called a temporal lobe epileptic, that he was given to seizures. I believe that's
probably true. Temporal lobe epileptics are disposed to have
religious visions. It's later in that fifth episode that we see the

reverend have a seizure for the first time. What we see in the second half of that season is the minister getting sicker and sicker with what the doc realizes must be a brain tumor. The minister is losing his mind. There's nothing to be done. The disease must simply progress. The reverend has to live through the changes. Everyone around him has to live into their inability to do anything to change the outcome. Ray McKinnon's work was something to behold. What was gone and what was left, in his body and on his face. He's gone on to write a wonderful show of his own.

HBO likes a whole season to be finished before a show goes on the air. That's different from the networks but suited me fine. We shot the first season from July 2003 to February 2004 and the show premiered March 21, 2004, two days before my fifty-ninth birthday. I like to keep saying my age to impress upon you that I was already pretty fucking old then, and yet somehow now I'm still much, much older. The final script of "Sold Under Sin," the twelfth episode of that season, is dated March 17, 2004, so that must be when we locked the final edit. I finish things when they're due. Then we just kept going, shooting from summer to spring, a little break between seasons then start again. For three years. It's very rare that one is given, in a work of that scope and scale, the opportunity to discover the rhythms and pacing that become the deeper, unsettled truths of the work. I was fortunate to be given by HBO the latitude to allow myself that. Obviously I owe a large debt of gratitude to the sponsoring organization, and in particular to Carolyn Strauss, who was the boss wrangler of our production, letting us find our way and believing on a weekly basis that a story could be told with the freedom that was afforded to our show, in the presentation of the lives of the characters and their experiences, to discover as we went along. It was an almost giddy freedom. One morning I got to the set at about 5:15, first dawn, and there was this owl that was always flying around then. He was looking down at me, and I imagined him saying, "You damn fool, what are you doing here at 5:15 in the morning?" And I answered to myself, "I'm doing just what I'm supposed to be doing."

* * *

The streets and sets were almost always dressed. The setup we had there at the ranch allowed us to work very organically. After a scene was written I'd go down on the set and we would walk through it. I would have my say and the director would have their say and the actors have theirs. I don't mean to suggest it's a democracy. It isn't. But I try to be respectful of what other people are feeling because that's the larger organism telling us something. Sometimes an actor doesn't do well with a particular kind of scene and I'll change the scene on the spot or I'll see something else going on that maybe we didn't realize was what the scene was really about. That's one of the upsides of working that way, everybody's prepared to change anything. Even in editing—I'd work with our great editor Elizabeth Kling—we could take the end of a scene and put it at the beginning. Move scenes around in an episode. She rigged a system so there was a black box I could look at when she had to scroll through footage, because the scrambling made me so crazy. She'd tell me, "Okay, look at the box while I move it." If you do a story with multiple points of view, if the form has multiple points of view, invariably the subject of your story must be man's encounter with the fact that there are forces outside his own sensibility that shape him, that the resolution of his experience will not be found within his own sensibility alone but in joining with those other points of view in common cause.

Toward the end of our second season Molly Parker came to me in some distress because she felt Alma's acceptance of Ellsworth's marriage proposal had not been adequately prepared for, and she was right. And so we were talking about it, about why she was making that choice, pregnant with Bullock's child, which she wants, and how now that child's needs mean she will have to declare herself someone else's possession, because that's what the world she's a part of asks of women who are to have a child. "Well, she needs to have this conversation with someone, but there's no one for her to have it with. Who would she talk to?" And then we thought, "Maybe it's Brom." Her dead husband, the man who brought her to the camp in the first place. "The conversation is in her head but that's who she's talking to, walking through the camp toward the graveyard." From that conversation I went off and wrote the scene, hearing Alma's thoughts:

ALMA (V.O.)

I don't know why I seek you out. If lying in the ground you can think or have feelings, you may hate me and my part in your fate as I sometimes hate you for bringing me here, though I know your bringing me was the end of something whose beginning I had as much a part of, certainly, as you. I am afraid. I am so afraid that my life is living me and soon will be over and not a moment of it will have been my own, and of how my body now tells me that is fine and right. Perhaps I confide to you because you cannot tell anyone.

She stops, still on the thoroughfare, not yet having left the camp—

ALMA (V.O.)

I am to have a child and I have a child in my care. He
is a good man.

She turns and starts back—

ALMA (V.O.)

And he whom I love is here as well.

All that came because Molly knew it needed to. Her performance of that scene had an urgency to it, the same urgency she
came to me with. The setting of *Deadwood*, the time period,
allowed us to more fully explore the complexities of being a
woman than a contemporary setting would have. We were able
to show in a very pointed way how women are conscripted to
their roles in this world, how at every turn their choices are
limited, and the question becomes how you might reconcile
yourself to it if you're not going to kill yourself. Alma, Jane,
Joanie, Trixie, Flora, Aunt Lou, Jewel, those are some very
complicated characters. There are stunted affects in each of
them because women are encouraged, often forced, to believe
that they exist as adjuncts of the male will or fantasy. Prostitutes were imprisoned in one way, women like Alma in upper-
class society in another way. Bustles and all kinds of strange
confinements. They were treated with this elevated rhetoric
that in fact was incapacitating to them. The word "hysteria" is
derived from "of the womb"—when a woman began to feel as
if she were thwarted she was diagnosed as being hysterical, the
diagnosis was literally that her womb was driving her. And they
would give her opium. Opium was prescribed for cramps, for
unhappiness, for anger—they got women loaded so they would

accept their continued imprisonment. Every woman character on the show had experienced one or another kind of sexual violence, as a child or an adult or both. On *NYPD Blue* we would sometimes get criticized that at some point every female character was either harassed or attacked or turned out to be the victim of child abuse or was pursued romantically at the workplace, that those things happening to every woman were over the top or unrealistic, as if that weren't the truth of a woman's experience in our culture. Which isn't to say we always got it right. I'm the product of a society in which women are not given the opportunity to develop as fully as men. It's always an admixture of the limitations of the artist's own imagination and the psychic cards that they've been dealt and the prevailing conventions at the time. I suppose too that on *Deadwood* I was working with more women. We were able to get to a fuller portrayal of the limitations placed on and violence done to women, and how friendships still form, how there are still ways to grab at more freedom, without necessarily knowing that's what you're doing, how heroic it is to still figure out how to be in the world at all.

The character Francis Wolcott was a pretty pure distillation of that violence. He kills prostitutes. When Garret Dillahunt finished his work as Jack McCall in the first season, we both wanted to keep working together. I knew Hearst was going to end up coming to the camp, and we talked at one point about him playing Hearst. As it developed, I realized Hearst would need to be more of a looming off-screen presence the second season, a fear, but he was going to send in his advance man Wolcott. This man would be one of the driving forces of the second season and Garret would play him. Some people were confused by that, the same actor coming back—I don't care about that stuff. I just know no one else could have played either of those parts like Garret did. He has a real protean gift. He is, more than really any other actor, hospitable to what is unprecedented in the sense of the character. It's not a parlor trick. He goes down and gets it. You can't be too cavalier about it, but there was also something in the soul of Jack McCall that reincarnated itself in Wolcott, a challenge to the community. They are both instances where the insistence on the illusion of separateness isn't just sad, it kills people.

* * *

I wanted to keep working with HBO and they wanted to keep working with me. We started talking about other shows we could do together in addition to *Deadwood*. I was thinking about this old *John from Elsewhere* script I had and HBO had been having conversations with the Fletcher family, this family of surfers. HBO put us in touch and asked if I thought I could combine those ideas. Mr. Rome-becomes-a-Western says, "Of course I can." And the idea of a wave was interesting, the wave as an expression of spirit. I got in touch with the novelist Kem Nunn, who had written a few very good novels about surfing and the border and Tijuana. The thinking was, we'll adjust the premiere date of the third season of *Deadwood* so we have some extra time for postproduction, and I'll rework the old pilot as a surf show, and a show about family.

We finished shooting *Deadwood* in maybe March or April of 2006. Kem and I get this pilot in. I was excited about it. I felt like there was a way to integrate a lot of ideas about commerce, about the internet. Never mind that I didn't really know how to use the internet, I saw the effect it was having on people. We were already figuring out the logistics of having two production offices at Melody Ranch. In my mind, that solved a lot of the problems we had had with *NYPD Blue* and *Brooklyn*

South—no traffic. HBO is excited too. They're so excited they want us to shoot the full *John* season before season four of *Deadwood*. And given that, the network reasons, it doesn't really make sense to hold the actors' contracts and pay the fourth-season option at that exact juncture. Perhaps better to let them out of their contracts and do other jobs in the interim? Now they're presenting this reasoning to me and my response is that this would effectively amount to canceling the show, that certainly that is how it would feel to the actors. Here is where the network asks me if I could conceive of doing the fourth-season stories in six or eight episodes instead of twelve. My answer at that moment, in whatever resentment I was feeling at my circumstances, was no. The network was not willing to do twelve. This is where the fact that Paramount still had foreign rights on the show was significant. That was a whole revenue stream that HBO didn't see a penny of on *Deadwood*. That it was a period show that cost about 4.5 million dollars an episode was probably also relevant. With a contemporary setting, I think HBO hoped *John* would be a cheaper show to produce. And so the option on the *Deadwood* actors' contracts was about to lapse, and I didn't want them to hear that from their agents.

I was still editing ahead of the third season premiere. I was in touch with the actors. Tim had just bought a new house, a few others were thinking about it. I called each one of them and let them know about the contracts, said we would still work on other solutions, but I didn't know what would happen and they should make whatever decisions they needed to make to best take care of themselves and their families. Those calls, that was one of the saddest days of my life. It was quite a wrench, the conclusion of *Deadwood*. It was unexpected and unprepared for. It's one of those days you're grateful you're sober because you don't know what you would have done if you weren't.

Chris Albrecht was head of HBO at that time. After the show's cancellation was already in the news, we tried to figure out one solution or another. Hours on the phone. I flew to New York. We announced that we would do two two-hour movies. Both hoped we would. Neither of us wanted it to happen the way it happened. But it did.

The consolation I tried to find when I wasn't busy being pissed off was that the idea of the end of a thing as inscribing the final meaning, the pressure that fixes the mark on the meaning of any experience, is just another one of the lies agreed upon that we use to organize our lives. You have to assume in some sense, the end of an episode is the end of things. The collaborative process of entertainment is itself a lie agreed upon—what you try to find is a coincidence of separate interests of art and commerce, and then sustain that coincidence for as long as possible, never forgetting the fact that the interests are separate. The moments of equanimity are achieved by submission of the self to the process of storytelling, which is the collective enterprise that I have found keeps me, most nights, out from under the bridge. Whatever the combination of corporate and personal imperatives that dictated the conclusion of the show, it's a child that believes those things go on forever and a child that believes you can never start over. I continued working with HBO and I continue to be grateful to them for working with me.

I know an awful lot of viewers felt betrayed and cheated by the abrupt termination of the series. Certainly everyone who worked on it did. It's also true that people try to allegorize experience so that we think we are tending toward some ultimate destination. Probably the biggest lie is the idea that we are entitled to a meaningful and coherent summarizing, a conclusion of something that never concludes. In that regard, what I told myself so I didn't set fire to anything was that *Deadwood*, the thirty-six episodes we did, was an engaging, sustained, imaginative experience. To waste time regretting or feeling betrayed as if there were some contract with the audience that was defaulted on, was to deprive oneself, as a member of the audience and a participant in the making, of the pleasure of appreciating what did exist. To attach bitterness to the encounter with what does exist is a failure of energy and truth. There was a lot of life there. At the end of it, to spend time regretting what might have been would be actually to distort what has been.

When it was announced the show was ending people hadn't seen twelve of the thirty-six episodes we had made. We were still in the editing room working on them. Sometimes I'd think to myself, "Geez, that's a nice scene. Boy, am I gonna miss this." And the "boy, I'm gonna miss it" takes me out of the scene. I've had plenty of time to miss it. But I only had a certain amount of time to work on the scene. The same discipline is asked of all of us. We were so privileged to do those episodes and it was such an uplifting experience, and we felt more when we were than when we weren't working on them.

The episode I was editing when I thought that was "Amateur Night," the ninth episode of the third season. The theater owner Jack Langrishe, played wonderfully by Brian Cox, in anticipation of opening his theater, hosts this amateur night where the people in the camp show what they can do, to make them more hospitable to the idea of theater. And so we've got hundreds of extras on the street, and I'm looking around for people to be a part of amateur night. There's this one guy, he's like five foot four, he's got neurofibromatosis, which they had once thought was Elephant Man's disease (what he really had was Proteus syndrome), and he's bowlegged. I'm talking to this guy and I say, "Do you got something for the show? Is there something like a trick or something you can do?" He says, "I have a rope-making machine." I said, "That's good. That's good. But something more involved?" He said, "I can cry at will." I said, "Now we've got a game." But I don't want him to have to speak. So I have him make a sign—"CAN CRY AT WILL"—and he holds it above his head. That's his act. Then there's another guy and I say, "Go over to him and say, 'I couldn't cry for my father when he passed away. I'll give you a dollar if you weep for him now.'" So we do that, then a little later in the scene you pan back, and the guy with the sign is sobbing, and the drunk who couldn't cry for his own dad looks at him and says, "'Course it's easy for you, you didn't know the cocksucker."

7.

Dogs and Cats

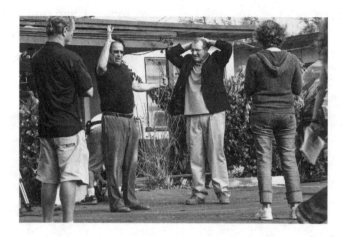

My tendency to become suicidally depressed when I'm not working, that alone gives some urgency to my getting back to work after a disappointment. Then add to that the idea that a few hundred people who worked on the production of *Deadwood* are also now out of work, and they don't have any development deal that pays them in the off-season, and I had told them less than a month before that I'd see them on set again soon. I'm gonna get going on this show quick. The strange twists of fate that led to the extra year or two of research on *NYPD Blue* and *Deadwood*, that wasn't gonna happen this time either. Whatever impressions I got, I had to get 'em fast. *John from Cincinnati* was, on its surface, about a family of three generations of surfers, like this Fletcher family HBO connected me with. The Fletchers were interesting, being the best at a thing for generations in a row, each time changing what people thought surfing could be altogether. Herbie walked on his board in a way no one else had. His son Christian was the first guy to do aerials on a surfboard, and he also had a drug habit which I found appealing. Dibi, Christian's mom and Herbie's wife, ran the whole show. Her dad and uncle had had a store that basically built the culture back in Hawaii. Dibi and Herbie invented and sold the tape that allows surfers to control their board in a different way. And Greyson, Christian's kid, who Dibi and Herbie raised, what he was really into was skateboarding, and he had this purity, and I wanted him to play the kid in the show. I met the surfer Keala Kennelly, and I asked her to be in the show too, as Kai. I met Steve Hawk, a surfer who had run *Surfer* magazine and gave his brother Tony his first skateboard, who then became a writer on the show. The thing I felt being around them all, and with Kem, was, "Whoa, this really is a different kind of energy. There's something else going on here." It all slows down a bit in a way that's kind of unsettling. And all of them, you get them on the water, or on a half-pipe, and they come alive in a totally different way. It's when they know best how to live, same as the bull riders. I remained obstinately pale and fleshy throughout this time. No one was getting me on the water. I don't even like sand on my feet. Maybe I should have paid heed to that, but I keep choosing to believe whatever happens is meant to happen.

Now, perhaps the bosses, whose original suggestion it was to incorporate this surfing family into the *John from Elsewhere* idea, thought they might be getting *Entourage* on the beach. But creatively, I had tapped into something on *Deadwood* and I didn't want to back away from it. By then, when we weren't at the ranch, we were at the Lantana building in Santa Monica and I was making friends with other writers. Guys like Jon Favreau and Judd Apatow, younger than me, really good at what they do. The way they responded to my work, and would share with me their ambitions for their own, it was exciting, it made me want to be bolder, or more perverse depending how you look at it. I had been reading a lot of Leibniz when I was thinking about and writing *John from Cincinnati*—that's why the character's last name is Monad. *The Monadology*, there are a bunch of different ideas in it that inform the work—substances being endowed with active and passive forces, the ability for a being to mirror the entire universe, and the movement of energy. It was this concept, the movement of energy, or the movement of a monad, that helped me to realize John was always supposed to be *John from Cincinnati* and take place on a beach. All energy moves in waves and particles, but the ocean wave is the only wave the naked human eye can see. If time is the lesson willing to be learned, the wave is time's expression. It comes again and again. It keeps saying, "Will you know me now?"

We were writing in 2006 and 2007 and along with surfing I was trying to wrap my head around technology and the internet (without actually using them much). Technology evolving exponentially fast, to what end? William James has this one book, *A Pluralistic Universe*, that compiles a bunch of lectures he gave, and he talks about this German philosopher Gustav Fechner, who basically believed that everything in the universe was alive and had a kind of mind. James built from that the idea of a compounding consciousness and the possibility of interpenetration between human minds and the mind of some kind of god and posited that "we may be in the universe as dogs and cats are in our libraries, seeing the books and hearing the conversations, but having no inkling of the meaning of it all." Even if we're pure rationalists, there's something about that idea that makes sense.

Every time one of our kids went to college, Rita and I got several more dogs. It was hard to tell from day to day how many dogs we had. We had a lot of dogs. One of the great pleasures in our lives in that period was watching the dogs array themselves in relationship to one another. Little dogs bullying big dogs because they were there first. Even as they sleep they have to be touching one another. Our oldest, Sam, was going blind, didn't have much more time, but he was the boss. Periodically, he'd bark to warn the other dogs: "I'm on post, believe me, do not try to get away with anything." We had this bulldog Frank. Absolutely the ugliest creature I ever encountered, had this underbite, but he was so self-possessed and so convinced of all of his virtues. The world was his friend and its proper role was to admire him. He'd waddle up to every stranger: "Go ahead, do what you need to do," and all were compelled to pet. He felt it his right for me to clean the smegma in the folds of fat in his face. He'd say, "Go ahead, Dave, go ahead." I'd take my finger, go to my wife, and say, "Smell this!" It was a joy for us, beyond even identifying with our species, to roll around with them and just watch them and talk to them.

Let's say that the Universe wants something from us. What the Universe wants, we don't know. It would seem to change a lot. If you anthropomorphized the Darwinian idea of natural selection, you could say the Universe keeps wanting life to manifest in different ways on earth. It may want something else somewhere else. If we are but dogs and cats in the universal library, that's what we are. I can testify that dogs are a lot of fun to watch, you see them fuck with each other, seem to be separate, sort themselves out as a united pack.

This idea of global warming and disaster and all that shit—to me there is such a fundamental confusion in the locus of the concern. People keep saying that if the ice caps melt, the earth is doomed. I don't get that. If the ice caps melt, a lot of people are doomed, maybe all of us, but there have been a lot of historical epochs where the ice caps melted and the earth seems to have done all right. We've only been around a little while. The odds are we'll be around maybe another two thousand years and then we're going to be gone and won't care about the ice caps. It's not that we can destroy the earth, we can't lay a glove on the earth. What we're talking about is the dislocation of the idea of human mortality and projecting it into the termination of the planet. It's arguable that all of this process of fossil fuels and the raising of the earth's temperature is just a way for the earth to get rid of us as pimples on the ass of its destiny. The argument that we should stop doing that is just one argument. Here's another argument you could choose to make—we should accelerate the process, to get rid of ourselves more quickly, and then earth could go back to that primeval, perfect place with tyrannosaurus eating brontosaurus.

If you anthropomorphize the earth as certain relatively respectable philosophers like Fechner have done, that the earth has its own will and mind, what you could say is that the earth is getting rid of us by coughing and putting all this stuff in the air. The earth is saying, "These people are too stupid." The idea of being concerned about the corruption of the atmosphere and smoking cigarettes, which a great many people still do, that begins to suggest a dichotomy between what rationally we understand is the good and the drives of our own nature. One thing that the earth could be saying is, "Interesting species, too aggressive." We say we've got the H-bomb under control. We've got chemical warfare under control. We've got nothing under control. We say that we've advanced tremendously from the time that we killed fifty million people eighty years ago during the Second World War and the tens of millions killed since. If you were a bookmaker, you quote any price—we're gone. Our technological advance so outstrips our emotional capacity to control the strength that we're giving ourselves as to give us no fucking shot.

So let's say that we're fucked and within being fucked there are certain aesthetically satisfying manifestations of our nature as humans. Surfing—physically pleasing to the eye, certain satisfactions of motion and symmetry. The people who are surfing, they seem quite fit, strong physical specimens. Can you extrapolate from that to some principle of governance? No. Nearly every one of them fucks up. They abandon their families or become monsters of avarice. The movements of grace do not translate into principles of governance, they're two different parts of our psyche. I had about fifteen interns at this point, some just out of college, some I had met in recovery, others that had come into the picture however. I don't say no to people. Or they don't even ask. I meet someone and say, "Come be a writer, work with me." Sometimes this is kindness and sometimes it isn't. A lot of them I hired when I still thought we were going to be working on *Deadwood*, which was a world I felt confident in, and then they're all there with me trying to find my way with this surfing show. That thing Swearengen does, where he looks at Burns and says, "How can you be that fucking stupid?" I did that sometimes. I could make them feel special, like they knew the world, then make them feel terrible, like they didn't understand anything. There was one day one of them was supposed to put a scene of theirs up on the screen for review and instead the guy was outside throwing up in the bushes. Scared to even show me his writing, didn't want to feel however I might make him feel. I was paying them weekly out of my own pocket, because I wanted to be teaching as I was writing and this felt like the right way. I paid for their lunch every day. Rented an additional office for them to work in. Lantana is a nice fucking office. Larry David down the hall. It wasn't cheap. At one point someone pointed out I couldn't afford all these interns, which I probably should have considered before hiring them, and I asked Bill to tell them all we would have to end the internship, to fire them, because I couldn't do it myself. The next day I hired them back. Maybe I doctored a script quick to get the money. I think we set a time limit on the internship then, that it would only last three months. Of course, it would have been more responsible to say that at the outset. Sometimes hating yourself is a fair response to the data. Let the fossil fuels burn, we deserve it. But for some reason I keep believing it would be better for me to be around people.

If you look at all the stars that have exploded, the combination of circumstances that produced life, as a matter of mathematics, it's one in at least twenty-seven billion or whatever, and yet it happened. What does that argue for? Nothing. It does suggest the kind of skepticism that can incapacitate us in our behavior. It's not that skepticism cannot be justified, but its existence, the fact of being skeptical—something can have more than one reason for being. We're not skeptical about the telling of this story because it's unlikely, we're skeptical about it because we are in a form of despair, which has to do with an absence of faith. What's the point of trying to teach when I'm enough of a sociopath that I traumatize the people I hire? What is the point of having a child? It's just going to die, right?

The argument of *John* was that the universe somehow cares about the outcome of our species' adventure, that it wants *us* to live. In a way that, as dogs and cats, perhaps we can't understand, the universe cares. We don't know how. We don't know why. It just feels like it cares. That may be our misapprehension. We're dogs and cats. At the level of content what we were trying to do was to have a spirit of the universe, the mysterious John, engage with the culture on its own terms, using its own language, and gradually persuade the culture to uplift its technology so that the species goes on. He parrots people's words back to them.

Ben was out of school for the summer and discovered this pit bull in a trash can that upon further scrutiny turned out to be a Great Dane that he bought at a pet store. This dog looks at you and his tail starts going, he'll go over and cuff the bulldog, "You like that, boss?" When he was still small, before we realized he was half Great Dane, I could conceal him completely in my hands. He had a lot of faith in something he didn't understand, in which sense I was his library. But also in his trust he made me a better person, and then I feel like I'm the one in the library again. John was like the Great Dane. At first you think he's dependent on these fuckups he somehow fell in with, that he doesn't know anything. But through being with him, we begin to identify John as somehow having a superior energy force. Here is a species that, in terms of understanding, seems to be less than us, but that we identify as possessing certain other qualities that are beyond us, and we like that. We identify with that. We feel that in ourselves as the best of us. All of the characters are so fucked up though at the start of the show, that even when they start to become better, when the miracle starts working on them, it's barely perceptible. Butchie goes two days without using, keeps talking about how he's gonna get dope sick, and he doesn't get sick. That's a miracle.

I wanted the fundamental challenge of these materials to be

the audience thinking, "What the fuck is this supposed to be?" I wanted the scenes themselves to be so radiantly specific that as you're watching them, you're so caught up in the confusion that you don't give a fuck, but afterward you're saying, "This is the last episode that I watch without knowing what the fuck this is supposed to be." Which is in fact the way we live our lives. "I've got to figure out what the fuck I am doing. Tomorrow is the day and that's the line in the sand, pal. Once I draw the line in the sand, believe me, tomorrow is the day." And then tomorrow goes by and it's the same thing. By starting each scene seemingly at the wrong time, you're really making the structural case for that approach. Which is that life starts where life starts.

The other quality that I wanted to get about the surf community is the strange relationship to youth. All these kids getting contracts at twelve years old. That's what the commercial culture would use the surfers and skateboarders for—to ally with that energy and associate it with youth before what they're really after becomes clear, which is commerce. The way that the dominant culture uses the surf and skate kids is essentially a form of pornography. The same way that you're marketing fornication in its most primitive form, you're also marketing the first movements of puberty, exploiting that energy and that strangeness. Actors who started working as kids have a similar experience. You've got these kids who aren't exactly men and aren't exactly women and you try to attach a commercial value to their youth. When those people get older, if they don't figure out a way to accommodate that experience of exploitation, they're fucked out. That's what happened to Butchie in our show. Looking around trying to figure out, "This was the good life, wasn't it? I did what I wanted to do, didn't I?"

We decided to set and shoot the show in Imperial Beach,

ten miles from Tijuana, right on the border. The impression I would always have in places like that is that the failure fully to have come into an identity is itself the identity. That's our folks. They're interrupted somehow. Without having been there, that's how I felt it would be. At the physical, geographical level, that setting is a readying for that story. It's almost like a moonscape. You want to shoot everything really wide. The other thing is not showing too much surfing or skateboarding, because every time you do, it should feel like this special release, this relief, and it has to feel precious, because that feeling is rare, and mostly inaccessible. Or what you have to do is interpose some obvious impediment to the viewer's appreciation of what's going on. For example, you only see thirty-year-old footage and the age of it dictates a primitiveness in the rendering that makes it obvious to the viewer that they're not getting the real feel of it. If he's seen from four hundred yards away. If he's one of six guys and then finally alone, but still a tiny figure. It's like when you're flying over the midlands of the country, and you're looking down, you are disabused of any idea that you really know what it's like on that farm down there. Rather than trying to get it right, you want to admit to getting it wrong. If I'm flying over these farms, when I look down, I don't get what being a farmer is about. But there is something about the magnificent futility of human endeavor in all that geometry that suggests an order to the universe, even as it's quite clear that it's not the essence of the lives that are being lived. When you see all those surfers crossing, it's like they're right for the wrong reasons. If I had more time on that show, I would have liked to cross the border more, shown the daily back and forth, maybe have had a guy who ran one of the booths at the car crossing, maybe a family that comes in in the morning for school and work would start coming to

Dr. Smith's clinic or Barry's theater once they opened. There was a scene in the pilot with the actress Rachel Ticotin in a jail cell with Cissy, Rebecca De Mornay's character, and Rachel in that one scene was able to suggest a whole life. I wanted to bring her back but I never got to it. I was writing as we were shooting once again.

We shot on location a lot, all staying at the Loews Coronado Bay. My old collaborators Gregg Fienberg and Mark Tinker were running the production. Maria Caso again doing our production design. You always want to work with people you've worked with before if you've had a happy experience. There's a shorthand that develops among people who have worked well together that is absolutely necessary if you're gonna do something out of the ordinary—you have to have faith in each other. The pure act of faith on the actors' part was extraordinary, because nobody understood what was going on, and they brought it anyway. Junie and Libby did the casting again, a mix of people I'd worked with before and some I'd never worked with and some like Greyson and Keala who'd never even acted before. Austin Nichols, who played John, had done two episodes of *Deadwood* as Morgan Earp, and Dayton Callie and Jim Beaver and Garret Dillahunt and Peter Jason and Paula Malcomson and Stephen Tobolowsky and Keone Young all came back around too. Willie Garson and Luis Guzman and Paul Ben-Victor, they had all done great work in recurring roles on *NYPD Blue*. Luis had played Martinez's dad and Willie had played a pain-in-the-ass tenant of Simone's and Paul had played Steve Richards the snitch who made me laugh so much. There was a scene in the fifth episode where Jim Beaver's character Vietnam Joe goes to the VFW bar because he thinks John was joking about his time in Vietnam and that means someone at the bar must have told John. Joe has all this shame from surviving, not saving his friends, and he talks to Ernie the bartender and shows a gun and Ernie says, "I never repeated your story to anyone, Joe. I don't believe you told us." In this convoluted way, it was John's strangeness that got Joe to finally tell his friend Ernie what happened. Ernie was played by Larry Brandenburg, who also played the bartender in the episode of *NYPD Blue* when Jim played Jesus the trucker. I was glad to have them together again, even if no one knew that. I don't even know if I knew that until they were on set together. And I was finally working with my dear friend Ed O'Neill again, playing a version of my best friend, Bill. Bill Jacks in the show helped raise and protect Shaun when Butchie couldn't, the same way Bill Clark helped raise and protect my kids. Bill's birds, Bill's sweetness with the children and birds, it's part of the first miracles.

I know it was easier for the actors I'd worked with before to proceed with the uncertainty of what we were doing, because they at least had past experience to draw on, which just makes the work of the actors who didn't have that past data a greater testament to their faith. Again I was interested in people who were very identifiable from a previous role as a way of mobilizing viewers' sense of the possible arbitrariness of how we remember things, tapping into their potentially fanciful associations with a performer and then scrambling them. I remember my daughter's response to us casting Luke Perry—she was sort of stunned with feeling and her own memories and I thought, well that's a wave. Mark-Paul Gosselaar and Jennifer Grey came on later too. Rebecca, Bruce Greenwood, Luke, Matt Winston and Brian Van Holt, Emily Rose and Chandra West, it was tough material, and they just kept coming at it. I was asking so much of them, I knew I was. I tried to do it responsibly but also didn't stop asking.

There isn't a lot of physical violence in the show, but there's a tremendous amount of emotional violence and degraded behavior. I wanted to show a family doing violence to one another. The violence doesn't mean they don't love one another, but that there is love underneath doesn't mean they aren't doing violence. Watching it, you wonder, "Why do I feel so brutalized? Nobody's getting killed." That's how anesthetized we've become. We forget emotional violence is violence even as we are responding to it. In the sixth episode, there's a scene where John realizes Cissy's about to kill herself, and he goes unconscious in the van with Bill and Vietnam Joe, then all of a sudden appears in front of Cissy's kitchen window. In Vietnam Joe's van they'd listened to a carpet store commercial and John picks up the rhythms and language of the commercial when he appears in front of Cissy:

JOHN

Are you sitting in your kitchen on Seventh Street, thinking of blowing off your head with your gun you got back from Kai's trailer? Have you completely run out of whatever let you put up with your asshole husband for thirty-one years? Do you feel that everything you ever touched in your entire life, you turned to shit and mud? Are you ashamed, Cissy, that once when Mitch was on one of his bullshit retreats and you were loaded on acid and Butchie was thirteen and he'd just won his first contest and you were so proud of him for not being Mitch, and you went into his room and he was whipping his skippy, that you said: "Let me show you how to do that."

John makes the jerk-off motion.

Have you wanted to kill yourself every day since, Cissy? And not even known it? And turned yourself into the worst ballbuster known to man, so no one would be with you, and you wouldn't have to be afraid that you'd ever do something like that again, that's how ashamed of yourself you were? Do you think now Shaun, who you loved so much and tried to make a life for, now you turned around and hurt his feelings so bad? Do you hurt so bad, you want it to just quit and be over? Everything? Well, let me tell you about our offer, Cissy. We prefer you don't. We wish you wouldn't. Our offer is: Keep going, feeling just as miserable, or worse. Hold the gun under the spigot and turn the water on. Spare Shaun finding you dead in the kitchen. And as a bonus, you'll also receive his love. Act now, Cissy. Baptize that fucking pistol!

And it saves Cissy. Austin Nichols brought such goodness to John, and Rebecca De Mornay's performance in that scene is wonderful—her gasp when he makes the jerk-off motion, when her deepest shame is out, you break with her, and you understand her. More of us than we'd like to admit have done something or many things that are absolutely shameful, have committed acts that have done real harm. If that just meant you were out, disqualified for good right there, the project of being a human would be much simpler. But that doesn't seem to be the game. It seems that we're supposed to figure out how to keep living.

The show went on the air in June 2007, two minutes after the last episode of *The Sopranos*. People were still very mad about the end of *Deadwood*. There were a lot of feelings to wade through before you even got to the show itself, and the show was challenging. It was confusing. The reviews were mixed. While all the reviews came out, we were still shooting, working on the last episode, and I knew the show wasn't gonna get renewed. Maybe even HBO said so explicitly, I can't remember, but I knew. And I knew the actors and the crew had read the reviews, and so this experience that was pretty tough already, the release they were holding out hope for, where people see it and say it's brilliant and they get to say, "Oh yes, we felt that all along," now they know that isn't gonna happen. Instead they're thinking the discomfort they've lived in for the last nine months is going to go on in perpetuity, a lifetime as a punchline, "What the fuck was that?" The temptation then is to start distancing yourself from it even while you're still in the midst of it. But we still have to finish. Our responsibility is to keep going. What do you say then? We were shooting the closing scenes at the pier with a few hundred people and someone had a camera that day and here's what I said: "Here's the thing. If you've fucked up unremittingly for decades"—I raise my hand—"you wake up and you say to yourself, how the fuck am I still alive? Don't they come and collect the license at a certain point? That's what the universe gives us every morning. No matter how far we have veered from reverence for the miraculous fact that we exist in a universe that we don't understand, until we stop getting to dawn, we get a chance to start over. The first episode was a starting over, and we have become so jaded, and so addicted, to wanting to be told what we are going to feel, that there's a certain withdrawal that one has to be willing to ask the audience to go through. Please know that I've never been prouder, or more grateful for the collective efforts of so many people, nor have I ever seen a more heartwarming result. So, we're kicking ass, and this is gonna be the culmination of it. Everything's gonna go fine." I take out some manuscript pages and start looking at them. "Now, having said that, there is no fucking script."

A few months after the show ended, our dog Stella got sick. She was a bit of a dim bulb so it was hard to tell at first that she was in distress, but finally it occurred to us. All the panting. Rita took her to the veterinarian and called me and said, "Stella's dying. She's got a tumor and she's in heart failure. She needs to be put down." I drove over there. When I went to see Stella before they put her down, I walked into the room and she looked at me and her tail started wagging. At some level she knew she was in distress, but she was happy to see me. I certainly knew she was in distress, and I couldn't bear it. I walked out. It is a weakness. I am a mere mortal and sometimes much less than that. Now we recur to our situation at least as we perceive it. Here we are: the victims of our own shortcomings. And here they are: the other, suffering our failures and reflecting them back to us. That is the distortion. That ain't what's going on. I knew that the blessing for Stella would be to be held and I knew I could count on my wife to do it. Because I think of us as sort of a unity, my wife and I, I was comfortable knowing that Stella would be held even if I wasn't sufficient to do it on my own. That feeling is available to us in our art. It's the essence of our art. The going out in spirit. The testifying to the going out in spirit by the act of imagination. And if we do anything less than that in our art, then we begin to posit ourselves as victims. That sudden onrush, that outgush of joy that each of us has experienced at one time or another, and probably posited as a mystery or a miracle, and certainly as transitory, is what comes from indwelling with that spirit which understands that our sense of separateness in every fundamental way is an illusion.

I'll tell you something else. Greyson Fletcher still skateboards. You can watch him on YouTube, skating around those bowls. Doesn't wear a helmet. There's this one video my daughter sent to Rita to show me. He walks into this crazy track or bowl or park or whatever the fuck it's called, and he gets an hour to learn the place and do a one-minute line. The first minute or two of the video, he's just riding around getting a feel for the space, falling, laughing, getting back up, touching different surfaces, seeing what moves and what doesn't. Then two minutes into the video, you see that he's got it, he's tapped in, and he goes batshit, doing things on his board that don't even make sense. The whole energy changes, you feel different, you know you're watching something that must mean something, but you can't figure out what. It's all still there.

8.

Three Stories

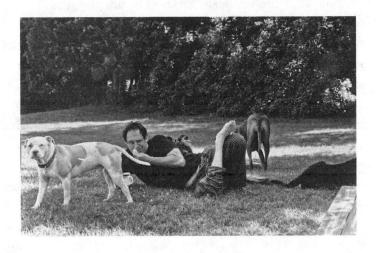

THERE ARE CERTAIN STORIES you keep going back to, that you think about for years and whenever you're asking, "What next?" you pick them up and dust them off and see what's there, if they hold your interest or especially the interest of anyone with the money to make them. It's Coleridge's categories of fanciful and imaginative associations again. Those stories that you keep going back to, there's usually a personal, fanciful association going on that keeps drawing you to it. The question is whether you can sink the roots deep enough to find the imaginative association underneath, the thing that will mean something not just to you in your fancy but to other people in its truth.

John ended in the summer of 2007 and the Writers Guild

contract was coming up for negotiation in the fall, but it wasn't looking like things would be resolved without a strike. Hollywood is still very much a union town, one of the few left. That's how we do as well as we do, which is still not even close to how well the bosses at the studios do. At issue in this particular negotiation were the residuals for DVD sales (no longer even mentioned in the official WGA history of the negotiations) and establishing residuals for airing and re-airing shows on digital platforms, which would prove pretty important. Every time the way people find art or content or whatever you want to call it evolves, it sure is helpful to have a guild making sure you don't get totally fucked. It only works if you all do it together. But anyway, the looming strike added a particular urgency to figuring out what to do next and turning a completed pilot script in before the deadline, because I wouldn't be able to for however long the strike went after that.

I always thought about something set at the racetrack, that was one idea. The first script I worked on when I was still teaching was a feature called *The Main Chance* set at the track. I wrote the same few pages over and over every day for a year or so. There was a seed image in my mind as I tried to write, which was hands paying money through a wire screen, but I couldn't see the rest of whoever's hands they were. I used to think, "If I could only see whose hands those are, I would know what's going on." I would fixate on that moment and write about it, and the extraordinary thing for us as writers is you come up with all sorts of ways to distract yourself from the idea that you don't really want to write about this. The hands were just the hands of the teller. Someone had to get their money and go back to their table. The story was about the people sitting at the table, but I kept staying with the hands to avoid the people at the table.

Then there was a story my brother Bob and I talked about a lot, which was the founding of Johns Hopkins Hospital. Bob's son Mike was a writer and he had come to L.A. and worked with me for a while, and this was one the three of us kicked around a lot and with a few other writers in the years to come. All three of us are drawn to that story, and the idea of working on that together, for personal reasons. My dad was in the hospital from his accident the first two years of my brother's life. There's some sense in which my brother was chasing after my dad his whole fucking life. He became a surgeon. He joined the staff in the same hospital our dad was on. My dad and my brother were on the same surgical staff. My dad never watched my brother do one operation. My dad was a little threatened by anyone he perceived as a rival. His uncles who were his peers, who his mom helped raise. For my dad, sibling rivalry was not restricted to brothers.

When my brother and I were young, he used to get us those Landmark Books that kids read. Ben Franklin, young fucking lightning rod. Bob would always find stuff about doctors because he needed very much to idealize. It helped him. The same image that I had, hands putting money through the window, that's a way that I had of not seeing what was nearby. The idealizing of the image of the doctor was what helped my brother, I suspect, not see the person who wouldn't wait up for him, wouldn't come watch him do surgery after all his years of working to get next to him.

So we're thinking about this series on how American medicine was created at the Johns Hopkins medical school, and as it happens, the great American surgeon was a guy named Halsted, who was also a junkie. The genesis of our interest came from my brother's and my fanciful, private relationships with our dad, with each other, with my nephew's fanciful associations with each of us, all of our associations with medicine itself, but if we do the work, the process of storytelling will ultimately erode what is fanciful.

It's probably safe to say that Halsted had some issues around sexuality and gender identity. He was an orchid raiser, big orchid raiser. He was married but he lived on the second floor and the bride lived on the third floor and the bride was rather an active lesbian. His OR nurse was also the woman who would smuggle his heroin to him while he operated. She came down with dermatitis because they used to dunk their hands in carbolic acid to disinfect and Halsted said, "I cannot operate under these circumstances." The real problem being he couldn't get his dope.

At the same time, a member of the Goodyear family got sick. This Goodyear wired back to the tire and rubber factory, "Make some fucking rubber gloves for this nurse so I can get my operation," and they did, and she wore them, and Halsted agreed to operate. That's how they discovered that if you wore rubber gloves, infection diminished.

Johns Hopkins himself was a Quaker whose father had a revelation that slaveholding was a bad thing. This was after the father had made about, in our money, twenty million bucks off being a slave owner. Better late than never. Johns Hopkins, he didn't own slaves, but he sold dope. He was a big liquor salesman, and tobacco salesman. A very pious man. So when he died, he left all of his money to set up a university, a hospital, and an orphanage for Black children. Those institutions therefore were properly the expression of impulses spinning against the way they drive.

A lot of Johns Hopkins's fortune, because he was a Baltimore boy, was in the Baltimore and Ohio Railroad. The railroad barons were all swindlers and thieves and stock manipulators. In that time there were several financial panics not dissimilar to the ones we live through now, and the only problem with the bonds these guys all held was they were worthless, but they're only worthless if you admit that they're worthless. If you can get somebody to buy them, then they ain't worthless. The inheritors of a large portion of these bonds were daughters of Johns Hopkins trustees.

In those days women weren't admitted. Coeducation wasn't going on, particularly at the graduate level. One of these women, Carey Thomas, her dad was a trustee at Johns Hopkins, she wasn't that pretty, and when she was a kid, regrettably she was set on fire, and it took her mother a couple of minutes to get there, so she was horribly scarred. Her mother was quite an accomplished woman. Her sister became a great suffragette, and Carey Thomas herself would wind up the second president of Bryn Mawr College. But she would never let her dad, who was a doctor, change her dressings. She made her mother do it. It was a kind of punishment for the mother not getting there in time. Also there were a bunch of other kids and this way she got her mother's attention. A lot of mixed motives. She became very active in her sexual identity at a time when lesbianism had a lot of euphemisms attached to it. There was a lesbian relationship that was described as a "Boston marriage." The sexual component of it was rarely referred to even by the people involved. Women just lived together. Not Carey Thomas. She was seducing women right and left, most of whom were more attractive than she and some of whom were also daughters of the other trustees of Johns Hopkins. She led the daughters in working out a kind of quid pro quo with their trustee parents whereby the daughters would provide the bonds that could be used to finish building the school in exchange for coeducation. And because the trustees also didn't want to admit that the bonds were worthless, they took them, and that's how women got into the school. It's all just variations in the extent to which you can get people to agree upon the worth of a thing from day to day.

The series of juxtapositions of accident and obsession and woundedness, that's how that explosion which began all of energy and all of life continues to compound and express itself. As I tell you about these people, you can see where that'd be a pretty fucking interesting story to tell how American medicine got invented. How revolutionary operating procedures came out of people trying to get their dope (always a prime motivation for me), how bad bonds and Carey Thomas sleeping around helped get women admitted to the school.

The third story was about my friend Bill Clark, about when he first joined the detective squad in the NYPD. Bill had joined the army at seventeen, in the early sixties, was sent to Europe for a while, then to Vietnam. He was a scout-dog handler, he still cries when he talks about his dog Mox. When he got back in 1969 he joined the NYPD, and they sent him undercover right away. They didn't let him go to the Academy so no one would make him, had him infiltrate the Young Patriots, which was part of the Rainbow Coalition with the Black Panthers and the Young Lords. At the same time, after Frank Serpico's testimony, in 1970 Mayor Lindsay formed a panel called the Knapp Commission to investigate corruption in the police department. Bill was undercover for two years, helped them make some weapons arrests that probably prevented a few bombings. When he gets out from undercover in '72, he's made a detective right away, in recognition of the work he did. The Knapp Commission report comes out at the same time, and one of the report's recommendations is to put informants in every precinct to help root out the rampant corruption that's been revealed. No one on the squad knows Bill because he'd been undercover for two years, and now this young kid makes detective, so most of the guys in the squad think he's a rat from the jump. At the same time, some members of the Black Liberation Army kill two police officers in the street for being cops. The department was so thoroughly demoralized at that time, but not just the department, everyone else too. Society in general, and the city as one part, felt itself to be imploding. All bets were off about everything. Nobody knew what the play was— about sex, how to get high, how you were supposed to dress. Nobody knew what the fuck was going on. The society of cops was just one version of that, felt they were being unfairly demonized, nobody trusted anybody. Young Bill, who'd spent years just wishing to be a cop in a straightforward way, no one would even talk to him. They wouldn't tell him how to fill out his forms. Our show was gonna be about, in the midst of all that, this kid still finding a mentor, and still finding his calling.

There's a version of being a cop, the essence of being a good cop is the same as the essence of being a good person: get to the particulars, learn the details, see people as individuals. But in a demoralized atmosphere, you don't do that. You say, "Fuck all of them!" A lot of cops were so demoralized that that's what they were saying, "Fuck everybody." But despite that demoralization, there are some people who go ahead and do the work. What we were trying to draw was a world where there is no reinforcement for doing the good thing except wanting to do the good thing, where everything else has fallen away. Where if on a single day a person does good, all he can say in his own private conversation with his god is, "I did what I believe you would have wanted me to do in this situation. I know tomorrow I have to start all over again. The fact that you gave me the gift of today doesn't mean I'm not a shitheel or that I don't have shortcomings or any of that." That's what Bill did, whether he knew it or not. When he retired, he gave a speech, before he started to cry like a baby, where he said, "Thank God for the guy who thought of this job, who gave me a place to stand where I could serve." You just try and help your brother and sister get through the day. With this new show, I knew you needed to see that in the kid's face before anything came out of his mouth, because what comes out of his mouth is gonna be confused, because he's bitter, feels let down by the country after his service, confused by what he had to do undercover and the Knapp Commission findings, but denies all of those feelings. Bill still struggles with that, but you look in his face and you realize he just wants to have done the right thing. Even now, if you watch him go in and put his hand out to his birds, there's still that quality.

His idea going in was, you join up to do good. Same as when he went into military service. And then he realized it was more complicated. There were good guys and there were bad guys on every side. The job is the same thing. With the show, which we ended up calling *Last of the Ninth* because it takes place in the Ninth Precinct in the East Village, you're telling the audience you're gonna find out what the kid finds out, which is, as much good as you want to do, it's not gonna come to you that easily. For an audience, "doing good" is to understand emotionally what the fuck is going on in the story. And what the show was saying was, you have to put in your investment before we trust you, before the other detectives trust you to explain what the fuck is really going on. Because until you've lived it, you can't really fucking know. I'm not saying that to defend cops or police. Cops have been hired by society to be in the foreground of a very oppressive apparatus that keeps different people in very particular positions. That is the job they are hired to do. Cops also know part of the job is to keep secret what they actually do to keep everyone in their particular position, and that if they don't keep it a secret, people hate them for it, and on rare occasions they might even be prosecuted for it. That's why cops only trust other cops. The countermovement of the series was to demonstrate that the only way a cop keeps his humanity within that agreement is by widening out his trust to even those he perceives as his enemies.

There were a lot of different characters involved with the Knapp Commission and the NYPD at the time and Bill knew many of them. That was a blessing for us as storytellers but also a challenge. There's the historical truth, the truths of Bill's feelings about his own life and the people he knew, and the truths of emotional coherence for our story, and sometimes we'd get caught up navigating those. We were also bringing out some other older detectives to tell their stories, and even forty years later, they're trying to decide if they can tell the truth, and we're trying to decide if we can believe what they tell us, or at least can find the emotional truth of what they're trying to tell us.

A guy who we didn't talk to but we talked about was Al Seedman, the chief of detectives from 1971 to 1972. Bill didn't like him, thought he talked up his experience too much, in particular on the Kitty Genovese case. But we were trying to figure out if as a character he could be of use to our story. The fact that this guy in real life maybe was a bit of a shitheel, or a taker, or in recounting his experiences he became grandiose or appropriated other people's work, I take all that for granted, with everybody. We would have detectives visit with us and say, "Oh, I didn't know anybody corrupt. No one I knew." They're lying. Flat out. Some lies we find forgivable depending on our connection to the person and some lies we find offensive. I am not suggesting or analyzing the worth of one guy as opposed to another. Nobody tells the truth. They tell a version of the truth with their emotional associations. Sometimes what someone ultimately is trying to say is, "Listen, I tried to lead an honorable life." But instead of saying that he says, "Nobody was taking." I have to understand what he's trying to say and discount the fact that, if I stay on the surface of things, what I could say to him is, "You know what? You're a liar."

* * *

We turned in a pilot script for *Last of the Ninth* the day of the strike deadline. Actually I sent that script in like seven minutes after the deadline. We writers are unlovely creatures under duress. We're no day at the beach under the best of circumstances, but I send it in a few minutes late and I'm thinking, "These miserable bastards, there's gonna be a grievance. I'm seven minutes late and I'll probably be brought up on charges." That's an index of my predisposition to project onto the other—whether the other is our ostensible leadership in the union or the bosses at the studios or networks—a malice and a kind of punitive attitude toward me which is at least four to five percent legitimate. With the strike going on, after the draft's turned in, I'm not supposed to write anything. I feel generally depressed because I have this very tentative, ambivalent relationship to order, to the structures within which I operate, and my bridge to the world just got shut down. All sorts of antisocial behavior occur as a possibility in response to that. So in an attempt to ward that off, and give myself something to do, and connect with my brothers and sisters who perhaps feel the same way, I rent the Writers Guild Theater to teach another class.

So there we were at strike central. I liked to think of wherever I was as central. My self-centered fear, the secret suspicion that I nourished or at least cohabitated with was: "I am very lucky that I have had any kind of employment at all—if they ever knew what's going on in my head, not only would I be unemployed, I would be institutionalized." Now, I have been, and it's okay, but that's jumping ahead. The sense of panic and disempowerment and desperation that I suspected was percolating in the consciousness or the unconsciousness of a lot of writers during the strike because we weren't working—I made those feelings, working through those feelings, a big part of the class. What I believe is that we actually have those feelings all the time, but the strike presented a particular opportunity to access them and look at them in the light.

We are asked to go out on strike. Maybe in that strangeness we say we hate our Guild leaders, or we love our Guild leaders and we hate the bosses. Our idea of those who legislate the order in our lives is wounded and distorted. When I talk to writers who are more or less within the walls of the city, they piss and moan: "I take notes from morons all day long and I have to do it because they're my bosses." But what I hear is: "I'm home. I get to do my work and I get to resent the organizing force in my life." The only downside with that is if they also say, "And I'm writing shit!" If that's the case, that's a form of despair. If you have to say that you're writing shit for whatever reason, you've lost the possibility of the bridge to the world that our art offers as a way back from our woundedness. If we have a stake in believing ourselves victimized, we pursue situations in which we can conceive of ourselves as victims. The resentment and doubleness and antagonism and apocalyptic resentment of order—the structures of art offer us an alternative to all of it. But we have to be brave enough, to let that participation heal us. All of us have had the experience, the flickering experience, of what art's possibilities are. For just an instant you feel whole. For just an instant you feel part of things. There's a wave that comes over you and you think, "I'm home, and nobody's trying to hurt me. I have a place in the world."

But back on strike, or dealing with the bosses, the writer is persuaded, "You're weak." Or just waking up, the voice I would hear went something like, "Oh! He wakes. Oh, that's his idea of urinating, with a split stream. That's how he thinks coffee is supposed to be made. Look, that's how he thinks the ignition of the car should be turned on." That's why I want to shoot up. What the writer hears from the bosses is, "You are a child. And I love children, but let's be frank. Let me do the adult stuff, and you be your nutsy, crazy, childish self. We'll give you some money. We will let you feel whole. We will let you feel as if you are within the walled city. You're not coming right up to the altar because that's a whole different thing. I can't even explain that to you because you are a child. But it's gonna be warm here, no more raw sewage out there and no more of that aching sense of apartness that you've carried even before you started to write." The AMPTG, or whatever the fuck their initials are, the studios and producers the Guild was negotiating with to decide what we'd get paid for our work when it streamed—what we hear them say is, "You don't understand what goes on inside the main room and we don't want to burden you because you have this other nutsy, crazy gift that we love so much, that you tell the stories. We have to make them endlessly replicable and you don't know how to do that because you can't even show up for a dentist appointment. So you let us be the bosses. Live in fear of us, and in return you are allowed to resent us. You can go home and say to your partner, 'These cocksuckers!' Push comes to shove, that's what you need, that's what you enjoy. Because you're never going to be other than a child, are you? Because we yelled at you at the dinner table." I'm projecting all of this onto all writers or artists or whatever because that's how I've always talked about it. Maybe it's just me. But I don't think it is.

In January 2008, HBO announced they had given *Last of the Ninth* a pilot order. The strike ended the next month. We went into revisions and casting, and we shot the pilot that summer on location in the city. Carl Franklin directed, and Ray Winstone and Jonah Lotan were cast as our leads. Ilene Landress, one of the great television producers who had run production on *The Sopranos*, oversaw the day-to-day. A lot of actors were doing such good work even in just a few short weeks—Lily Rabe, Kevin Rankin, Michael Raymond-James, Brian Tyree Henry, Michael Gaston, David Moscow, Maddie Corman, Raphael Sbarge, Chance Kelly, Fredric Lehne. Then you edit and you wait.

In January 2009, HBO announced they weren't picking the show up. I hadn't had that experience in a while, and never before with HBO, but I was very fortunate that I still had my deal with them, and they still seemed to want to work with me, so I decided to think more about the horse-racing show. You can't know what would have been otherwise, if at that particular moment I'd ended up working on a show that put me back with Bill or with my brother Bob, instead of on my own at the races. But as it happened, I started going back to the track more regularly.

9.

Zenyatta

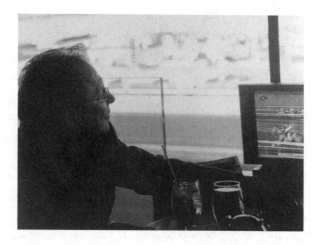

THERE'S A LINE AT THE END of *John from Cincinnati*, where Ed O'Neill's character is talking to his dead wife, trying to describe to her what happened over the last week, essentially over the show itself, and he says, "Where do you start and stop? Every event and incident . . ." That's how I feel trying to explain what happened when I started going back to the track, and working on *Luck*.

I've talked a fair amount now about the process by which art can transform the meaning of the past. The hope going into this work, not fully articulated but nevertheless moving in me, was that through the art, my experiences at the track would be transformed, would come to mean something new. That had happened to me enough times that I believed it was possible. I still believe it's possible. But that wasn't what happened this time.

The track is such a rich world. The characters and setting, the beauty and majesty of the horses and, on the deepest level, the purity of the connection experienced by everyone watching the race for that minute and a half, even while everything outside of that minute and a half, and even some of the things within it, are distorted in any number of ways—that's rich ground to till. I was compelled to tell this story for a variety of reasons, not least of which was my own cultivated and nurtured identity as and commitment to being a gambler.

My very problematic and uneasy relationship with the past and its connection with my present had historically had its negative expression in my being a heroin addict. One tries to find, to the extent one is a little bit imprisoned by one's past, benign accommodations to express that connection. *Luck* was an attempt at one such accommodation. Gambling and horse racing were inextricably associated with my relationship with my old man. The most time we spent together was at the track, sometimes also in the company of the man who sexually abused me, and almost always with my dad's ongoing narration of my degeneracy. That association came to inform my idea of relaxation, or enjoyment, or success. Ask my kids what it was like to go with me to the track, and they'll tell you it wasn't fun, or at best it was fun intermittently. They liked seeing the animals at the barn, and learning how to read the racing form so they knew who was the long shot and who was the favorite. But my eldest also describes being five years old, speed walking to chase after me through the clubhouse trying to keep track of me as I went to the booth to bet, not running because she didn't want to draw anyone's attention even though I was moving that fast, thinking, "I've got to keep my eye on him, because he sure isn't keeping his eye on me." Rita eventually started taking her own car when they did come, so she and the kids could drive home separate from me. When you win a race, they take your picture in the winner's circle. Almost every picture we have where the kids are there, we're all grimacing, because we just ran through the track and I was yelling at them to hurry the whole way. At the same time, they knew if they made it through the day, I'd give them a couple hundred dollars at the end, and they liked that part too. We had a drawer in the dresser in our bedroom where I kept cash and race tickets. Sometimes there'd be hundreds of thousands of dollars cash in there. Each of my kids learned to steal with that drawer. They'd show it to friends who came over. It was one of the fun parts of our house, like having a pool but harder to explain. You pass on some lessons whether you want to or not. But making them chase after me was maybe also my way of telling them they didn't belong there. They weren't like me in that way. I found a way to say that too.

It's useful to think about what's involved in the process of gambling in its connection to Las Vegas, which is a much more comprehensive and straightforward symbol than the racetrack. Horse racing would never admit it, but Las Vegas has been one of the deaths of the sport. Casino gambling provides the ability to gamble beyond time, rather than the particular moment of a race, and of course doesn't have the inconvenience of having racehorses. The race itself, the creatures, the shared event, there's something there that still insists on life as lived in time, and casinos go beyond that. You can't find a clock in a casino. The difference between night and day, it's very hard once you're in the casino to see the outside. When you go to Las Vegas, that city is organized intentionally to obliterate the disciplines of time. The entire environment is contrived to assault the individual sensibility with the symbols of the American definition of success and to make accessible the most garish versions of the American definition of success, absent the constraints of time and history.

The ad campaign, "What happens in Vegas stays in Vegas." That's not self-evident. It's a fiction that suggests, "Whatever you do in the real world, don't worry about it. You can come to Vegas and reinvent yourself and here are the instruments for reinvention. Craps, pai gow, slots. Talk about a range of possibilities! You can either be a pai gow degenerate, or you can be a slot degenerate. It's not like you have to confine yourself to one thing. You stay up, you don't have to sleep. The food's right here, if you happen to remember you're a creature who eats." That is the embodiment of a system gone mad, which has recognized that human beings can be made to want anything based on association. As long as you have the symbol agreed upon, which is currency, you can be a part of a self-sufficient and perpetual alternative reality.

Why do I shoot dice? "Seven! Seven a winner! Seven a winner—ooooh! Mister M, Mister M." That's all that there is. You never keep the money, but it's a moment when the world recognizes you, "Mister M, seven a winner." You become addicted to "Seven, a winner, Mister M." The only way that I'm a winner is if I roll a seven. The corollary of that is, "Oh Christ, if I could only roll a seven, I might be a fucking happy man. I'll tell you something, if I were happy, I would help a lot of people."

As long as you're winning, you don't care about time, but the moment that you run out of the currency that entitles you to admission to the world, you're out, and back in the time you wanted to leave. The house is there forever. The house has inexhaustible currency, and you're there only as long as you can play within the rules of the game, which is as long as you have dough. Ultimately, since your energy is not inexhaustible, you're going to fuck up, and you're going to be out. People who have had that experience sit around with a kind of stunned, vacant look in their eyes asking themselves, "What just happened?" What happened was they were exposed to a false environment, an environment that reorganized the categories of reality, which seemed to deny the dominion of time, and whose predicate was ultimately revealed to be inimical to the human spirit.

We can take a step back and compare that artificial environment with the artificial environment of art. Art is also a reorganization of the categories of reality, but one which, when responsibly executed, pays tribute to time in its relation to the past and the relation between past and present. Time is lost in the literal sense, but to the extent that the storyteller is responsible and humane, time is reintroduced as a theme, and to that extent the experience for the participant is a "responsible" kind of escape, as opposed to the kind of obliterating, apocalyptic escape that's involved in gambling.

For me, the association of gambling, or particularly the racetrack, with freedom or success is purely private and fanciful, having to do with my early relationship with my dad. There is nothing freeing or fulfilling inherent in gambling. Quite the opposite. It's a corrosive process that undermines one's humanity. The environment of gambling negates the sense of human connection—the kind of purchase price that you pay for entering into that world is an allegiance with the disciplines of that world rather than with human connection, making your own child run after you so you can place your bet just before post. The casinos and the racetracks, in reorganizing reality to exclude time, undermine the individual's resources in relation to the experience. It erodes the individual's ability to sustain relationships with the past in a healthy context, it stunts your coming freely to the present and opens the door to a sterile kind of reenactment of whatever crippling relationship one has had with the past. If you find yourself in pursuit of that reenactment, and also find yourself continually and further distanced from what you feel is the satisfying and correct configuration of that reenactment, you pay a price to stay in action.

I was fortunate to achieve material success in my career. But my material success was a convenience, it wasn't a purpose or a goal. Money wasn't the point. It was a requirement but it wasn't the purpose. You can try to use generosity as an antidote to self-hate. If tips didn't feel like enough, I could try to accommodate my impatience by offering promises to be collected at a later time—"mortgaging the future to save the present," as my wife would describe it. To the extent that I'm an unreliable person, I'm hypersensitive to acting like a reliable one. My deepest belief about myself is that given half a chance, I'll steal your dope and help you look for it, so I try to be rigorous going against that. A waiter wants to be an actor, I sign them up for acting classes before the check has come. Someone's mother is sick, I insist on paying for the hospital bills, or the funeral. When a gambler comes into some money, they say, "We'll let him hold it for a while." That's the same way with getting rich.

There was a time when I was making five million dollars a year, but the fact that I was losing five million, in his heart of hearts, is what would have made my dad proud. There was such a powerful impulse toward annihilation that was consistent in him. I remember him sitting with me once trying to work through when I had sold my novel to three different publishers or some other insanity, "What the fuck are you doing? What the fuck are you doing?" Finally he looked at me and said,

"You're no fucking good," and that's when I knew he was proud of me. My father was proud of what others might have identified as demonic in me. Insofar as *Luck* was inspired by my associations with him, it is fitting that though an honorable effort, the process of the work itself involved an annihilation of the spirit.

So what the fuck happened?

I wrote the pilot in 2009 and was going to the track more throughout that year. HBO liked it, but I suspect they were also trying to figure out a way to get me a bit more under thumb, not rewriting things on set, which cost money. The script was sent to Michael Mann, and he ultimately came on to direct the pilot and as an executive producer as well. Part of his coming on was an agreement that he would have final say over casting, and on set, and in the edit room. I agreed to all of it, even though it was very different from the way I had grown accustomed to working, and different from television generally, where the showrunner, the final boss, is usually the head writer, rather than a director. But I also knew I had had a few misses, and I think I felt compelled to show everyone I could go along to get along. It wasn't lost on me that Michael had made a great deal of wonderful art and that someone with his level of skill could do likely revolutionary work with the racing scenes in particular. People seemed excited about the prospect of our working together. It made Dustin Hoffman interested in being a part, and Nick Nolte and John Ortiz and a number of other great actors.

We shot the pilot in April of 2010. It was not a happy collaboration for me. Michael insists upon a single voice, especially on set. I couldn't go to the set, literally I was forbidden from going. That was a loss. If we're going to engage with him as a reality, then it behooves me to evaluate him, and I don't want to evaluate him. He's a driven, enormously articulate figure, but when I watched the pilot, there were moments or sequences where I thought he was wrong. Had I been directing the series, it would have been a different series. I don't think he knew enough about the world he was trying to portray. There are certain distortions that are his idea of the conventions of the story rather than the truths of the characters and situations. The last part of my writing is being on the set and working with the actors. I wanted the actors to live in the rhythm of walking with the goat, having the rooster around, feeding the horse a carrot. The animals are the measure of the true gentleness—the capacity for gentleness. It's being around the animals that changes you, but I wasn't there with them, so I couldn't insist on that, couldn't see what happened in those moments. Not being in the editing room, not getting to see all the footage that was there and other discoveries that might have been, that was tough too.

After the pilot there were some real conversations about how we would continue. We all still wanted to do the show. At one point, we were discussing a different potential future project of Michael's but also about how we'd work together going forward. We were talking about what soldiers bring to and take away from battle. I said to Michael, "When your mother fell ill, was there any fucking question where you had to be?" He said, "No, of course not." And I said, "Don't say of course not. For you." For Michael, if your mother is ill, showing up at her bedside is a given. That's a good thing, but that's not true for me. I don't see any human behavior as a given. And that's just one way we see stories differently.

In July HBO announced they were picking up the show and then throughout 2010 and 2011 we were writing and shooting. I know there's a story that Nick Nolte told of me taking a bat and saying I was going to kill Michael. I don't remember that.

But I remember feeling pretty fucking angry when I was waiting to see an edit. I felt so cut off from the process of the work. There were days I drove home and while I was at a red light I told my steering wheel, "This guy is an asshole and he hasn't lived very much." That kind of statement, ad hominem, ultimately diminishes the speaker. I know that. And yet I don't want to be perceived as bending over backward to avoid a fight. That was the question then, and in deciding how to talk about this it becomes the question now. At this stage in my life— old—I don't want to present a crippled version of my voice in order to defer. It's a pain in the balls. A moment has to come when you say your piece. But at the time I determined that bending was something I was going to have to live with. And while I couldn't be on the set, I could be in the clubhouse. I could still take people to the track and bet.

To better understand some of our characters who were also degenerate gamblers, Michael asked me what I felt when I won. I told him, "Nothing. Absolute contingency. Everything is at risk and the specific outcome doesn't depend on my character flaws, so that's a release." With our writers, I would describe what was going through my head when I went to the track to bet. " 'I'm going to drive out to the fucking racetrack. I'm going to bet starting with the first race. These are the odds and this was the horse's last two results and here's who the trainer is and here's how this horse does on this turf.' I'm distracting myself from what addicts call the committee, which would be berating how I stand and eat and drive and breathe. The committee is always in session and very personal. And the thing that I know when I'm not within my addictive run is nothing I can do is going to shut them up. But if I can submit myself to an artificial environment, I can feel something else, and all I have to do is bet all the money I have. I have to risk my family's welfare, I have to risk every fucking thing, risk the humiliation afterward of 'Here's a guy they say has made over a hundred million dollars in his life and may wind up under a fucking bridge.' But there's a chance I could win and if I win for about an hour and a half I get to give the money away to people and feel okay about myself."

* * *

In the fourth episode of *Luck* there was a storyline about the running of one of the horses whose excellence we've come to understand and anticipate. The writing of this episode coincided with the real horse Zenyatta's performance in the 2010 Breeders' Cup, her final race. Going into that race, she'd never been beaten. The idea of the horse retiring undefeated has an enormous appeal which ultimately, I think, does a disservice to all of the deeper connections generated among the people who are privileged to participate in the horse's career, as a trainer or owner or even simply as witnesses. If you identify the emotion that one feels in the aftermath of a horse's victory, how do we interpret the emotions that come to us in the vicarious appreciation of that sort of performance? The impulse is to feel, "Well, I've now been associated with unalloyed, unqualified excellence." The trainer Charlie Whittingham used to say, "No one ever killed himself who had a good two-year-old in the barn." I don't know if he borrowed that from somebody else but what is implied is the idea of the beckoning future. Fitzgerald spoke of it in *The Great Gatsby* when trying to imagine what the first settlers felt the first time they saw the New World: "For a transitory enchanted moment man must have held his breath in the presence of this continent, compelled into an aesthetic contemplation he neither understood nor desired, face to face for the last time in history with something commensurate to his capacity for wonder." A scene or an animal can seem to embody and reward and fulfill everything that we imagine about the promise of life. As time goes on problems show up and some of them are inherent in that promise.

The day of the Breeders' Cup, I watched Zenyatta being brought over from the barns. Everyone knew this was the filly's last race, and so many people had a sense of identification with her, a horse who so utterly and wholly embodied excellence, and transcended in her excellence every limiting category, including the category of gender. What everyone knows and takes as a given in racing is a filly doesn't beat the boys. But she beat the piss out of the boys—it just wasn't an issue. The thing about Zenyatta was not only that she was a girl who at the end was running against boys, but she always let them get ahead of her first, so in effect she was always conceding luck as an important variable to the possible outcome. No matter how good she was, if she had enough bad luck getting around horses, she wasn't going to win. The more variables one can introduce and still sustain that sense of absolute indomitability, even as one is brought to experience with absolute certainty that the sense of indomitability is an illusion, the more precious the illusion becomes. So I was watching her being brought over and, inexplicably to me, when she knows she's going to run, she begins to dance. With a joyful sort of anticipation, and it seemed in some measure responding to the appreciation that she felt, she started to dance as she moved, and it was a kind of unabashed embrace of the pure joy of what she was and what she was doing. As they were leading her to the saddling area there was such an outpouring of appreciation and emotion and adulation, from the owners the Mosses who were walking with her and the trainer John Shirreffs, a good guy and a war hero. They all three understood the nature of the transaction, of the spiritual and emotional transaction that was involved with the people that loved her. They made her accessible. People were too close to her as she was being led over, and everyone was screaming, but rather than being held back, the witnesses were enlisted by the trainer and owners in a respectful demonstration of feeling. The more they were cheering, the more she was dancing.

As the race approached and she went into the gate, the thought that was coming to me was, "Don't let her break badly this time. Because she's got everything against her as it is, she doesn't have to get left too." When they broke, she absolutely got left, as was her wont. Typically, watching that filly get left, there was almost a perverse gratification, "Good, now she's going to show just how much better she is than them." Despite the liabilities of time and experience, knowing this was her last race, one allows oneself to hope, "Let her get the best of it." But she didn't. It seemed like she couldn't get hold of the track. Then, as the race progressed, she began to enact exactly the same course that she enacted in every one of her previous races. She was unutterably far behind, but then she began to move. She even saved a little bit of ground before the far turn, which typically she didn't do, swinging wide. The jock had to wait a bit before he got out, but once he did, at the head of the stretch, it looked as if she had enough ground still left to run that she could make it. And she closed beautifully. It took her a little while, it looked to me, to get her to switch leads, but she had a dead aim on that horse. I really started pulling for that filly the last eighth of a mile, even as one had the sense that it didn't look like she was going to get there. You start breathing in the rhythm of the horse, your body moves with her. As I'm pulling for her I remember, even from her last race, that that flickering doubt was one of the last and best ingredients of the experience of watching her run. Every time you thought, "Well, she can't get there," you felt too, "So when she does, it will be that much more wonderful. And it's her last race."

She didn't get there. One more jump. They said she was only beaten by three inches. The horse that beat her is a very, very good horse. That's what he is, and he needed every bit of racing luck that he had to put him at an advantage against her.

Afterward I was bawling like a baby and had been from the head of the stretch in a sort of inextricable association of feeling appreciation for her performance and gratitude for the opportunity to feel that appreciation. It seemed to me in the aftermath of the race, the last gift which was given had to do with the separation of that feeling of appreciation from the illusion of invincibility. That the final and deepest gift she had to give was the opportunity to accept all the qualifications of our finitude without having that dilute or alloy the joy that she made available to us. In other experiences, if one is lucky, we get that same last chance to distinguish between what joy comes to us and what I imagine is the laughter of the gods. William James said that after any victory, "something permanently drastic and bitter always remains in the bottom of its cup." It took all of her races and the conclusion of her career to come to the last draught of what was in the cup. To realize still, that in what one experienced as drastic and bitter for a moment was the final essence of victory as allowed to us to experience it. The victory was in the flowering of humility as the last of the feelings that she had made available. I remember a piece of literature once talking about the chance to live life all the way up. Part of living it all the way up is that experience of limitation.

As she was coming back, the jockey Mike Smith was absolutely devastated. Jerry Bailey was trying to interview him and Mike tried to say something back after Jerry said, "How do you feel now? How do you feel now?" Mike said, "I'm just trying to keep it together." Then he started to sob. To his credit, Bailey ended the interview. At the press conference later, Mike just absolutely broke down. He said, "It was my fault." Certainly that was an understandable reaction. It gives us a way to deal with the experience. We can appropriate it and say, "If I had done something different, then I wouldn't be experiencing what I'm experiencing now." But Mike knew, and everyone knew, that she had done the absolute best that she could and this was the outcome. Finally, what one is left with is the feeling of the magnificent irrelevance of the fact of her defeat, how absolutely irrelevant her defeat is to the experience that she gave us for all that period of time. The proper coda for the story is the people honking their horns as they left the track that day, just saying, "Thank you."

I had had that feeling at the track before with a horse named Gilded Time. Around the first season of *NYPD Blue*, I spent what seemed like a lot of money to buy him but it wasn't a lot of money for the horse he turned out to be. The reason there weren't too many bidders on him was because he was straight in the pastern, and the pastern absorbs the shock. What looks like the horse's foot is not the horse's foot, it's the horse's middle toe. And if you now imagine yourself running, and all of your weight coming down on your middle toe every time, you can imagine that a kind of shock absorber is an important thing to have, and an angled pastern absorbs some of that shock. A horse that's straight in the pastern, the shock goes up its leg in a more direct way, and most horses will protect themselves, but a really great horse, if he's sort of born to run, runs as hard as he can, even if the shock is going up his leg. So virtually every time Gilded Time ran he hurt himself, because he would not be qualified in that regard. And that both liberates the capacity for adoration and, if we are humble enough, reminds us that the feeling of being in the presence of excellence is an illusion, but it's the most wonderful illusion to have. It's the same sort of illusion that if we are blessed with children, or if we are blessed to love someone in a wholly satisfactory way, the impulse to associate the feeling that comes to us with the world being in a perfect configuration is almost inevitable. When you see a baby, you feel that whatever tragedy may ensue, at that moment tragedy is a stranger. The longer that we are able to sustain that sense of the horse's transcendent excellence, the more we become aware, if not consciously, that it is an illusion. We feel joy simultaneous with the sense that our joy, for all its genuineness, is predicated on a feeling which life will not sustain.

There is a sort of magical thinking that goes on leading up to the race by which we try to accommodate our human shortcomings in the anticipation of a union with excellence. You'll watch people at the horse races and as the race is about to start they're smacking themselves in the head and going through eight thousand idiocies as a way of accommodating their own human frailties, because they're so excited about the experience yet to come. After one of Gilded Time's early workouts, my trainer Darrell Vienna had said to me, "We got a whole new set of problems." When the horse was about to run for the first time, he got to the gate and I was going through this whole litany of self-defeating negativity. The gates opened and he was fifteen lengths behind. He just walked out, looking around. I started in on Darrell, "Goddamn it, how many times!" Darrell put his hand on my arm and said, "Watch." Before they even got to the turn he had gone past everybody and he was still doing the same thing. He was looking around saying, "Is this all you got?"

With the race in the fourth episode of *Luck*, I wanted the

viewer to participate in that part of the experience. Nick Nolte played the old man trainer Walter Smith, and Kerry Condon played the young jockey Rosie, and they both love this horse and along with the viewer they've been waiting four episodes for it to run a race, but they're also scared. When the gate opens and the horse gets left you are disabused of the idea that this is a super-horse, that nothing can stop him, and begin anticipating potential disappointment, "Okay, so he's going to lose his first race and then he's going to be a great horse." Then as he starts to move, "Oh! In his first race he's going to fall? What the fuck?" Those are all self-centered appropriations. By anticipating the outcome, we're trying to protect ourselves. Then she steers him, and suddenly there opens up an unimpeded path. The question becomes, "Is he good enough?" Then the answer becomes clear, he's good enough in spades. As the horse comes through the stretch you see everyone's heart open—Walter and Rosie and everyone else watching—having experienced all the protective strategies that we use to insulate our spirit from the defining limitations of objective experience. As one by one those limitations fall away and you become part of the collective perception of this creature, you realize, "It's just what I hoped for, except better!" You just start laughing, because it's perfect.

Every time a good horse of mine would go on the track it was just pure unalloyed dread because I'm in the presence of this excellence and I'm overwhelmed with how profoundly corrupt and degraded a soul I have. The question becomes, how is fate going to reveal the impropriety of my connection with this excellence? What one of twenty-five different ways is that going to happen?

In March of 2011, around when I was working on writing the eighth episode, our then business managers got in touch with Rita to encourage her to transfer the title for our house on Martha's Vineyard to our children. We had hired them back when our children were born because I couldn't be trusted, and whenever we were going to spend money, Rita would ask them if we could afford it. They managed the kids' tuition, the payroll at my company, credit card bills, taxes, the acting classes I paid for, the other tuitions and hospital bills and apartments I took care of for various people I crossed paths with. They had never raised any flags with her before, so the title change seemed strange, and Rita asked them to meet. She went into their office the next day, and they told her I had spent about twenty-three million at the track in the last ten years, and a lot of that in the last two, and between that, five million in unpaid taxes, a few mortgages she didn't know about, and the business managers' own fees, we were seventeen million dollars in debt. Rita then asked them why they didn't pull the alarm to her years ago. They said they were afraid I'd fire them if they did. When I was a heroin addict and Rita and I were dating, she would come home and I'd say, "You're not going to believe this. They robbed us again." I was selling the furniture. "Something happened." All of that stuff. Sometimes we are blessed with what they call a moment of clarity, and one day I was looking at her and she was nodding and I recognized that she weighed about eighty-five pounds because she was a codependent and as I was getting sicker she was getting sicker with me. And yes at some level being a dope addict saved my life because it routinized a kind of chaos, but that really didn't speak to the deepest truth of the situation which was, "I'm killing her." As I've told the story within various anecdotes, with whatever transient charm, you may have been able to feel, "Oh, that's just a kind of shorthand." But when I linger to look at her and see that she was dying with me, it takes on a different dimension.

Then think of her leaving books for me like she's throwing meat into a cage. She has such an enormous imagination, which often tries to be invisible or unobtrusive. Usually someone in her situation has been devalued or minimized somehow as a child, and the way we deal with that is to internalize it and say, "It's because I'm no good. I don't feel anything." But once you have one strong emotion, it can turn into love. What you initially love is your capacity to feel, and then who you're with when you're able to connect to your feelings. Sometimes you need to be with someone so wounded and so self-enclosed that it prompts you to try and overcome your own self-enclosure. She understood what the circumscriptions of my spirit were, and she dealt within them. With our children, she was able to behave with a full range of devotion and expression. And they're so good and so happy and that was her. Through them, I got to see her come into the recognition of her own positive presence. And now she had learned how thoroughly I had put them all at risk.

If you look at my behavior, that ambivalence toward order, toward reality, it proves out. The hotel room with the credit card I never paid. Selling my novel to multiple publishers. I don't believe money is real. I made whole shows about that. But what you believe about money is real. Money had been one way that Rita and my kids felt safe, that I helped them feel safe—generally there weren't too many ways I did that, and now that was gone. When she got home from the accountants that day, she had her steam-rage silence going. She handed me the list of payouts to the track. I looked at her and said, "Why are you showing me this?" I couldn't bear to talk to her. I said I was sorry and went to bed. Elizabeth was coming home that night for a visit, bringing her then boyfriend to L.A. for the first time. I hid for the first two days they were there. You think this is going to be the moment they realize what you really are, and they're going to turn away. But that's not what happens. They call you down to dinner and then you're all back in the kitchen together, and you keep going.

I kept working on *Luck*, but I didn't tell anyone what was happening. I couldn't go to the set and now I couldn't go to the clubhouse either. Rita called my psychiatrist and told him about the money. I likely would not have told him on my own. With my doctors I am usually well mannered but often evasive, which doesn't necessarily help them succeed in my treatment. But with the new context, my psychiatrist put me on Suboxone, an opioid substitute, to help dull my urge to gamble. That treatment didn't reach any of the fundament of what was going on. In a very ham-handed, intrusive way, it pointed me toward the necessity of mobilizing my denial and suppression. I became much more an actor playing a part, and it so happened the part I was playing was my life. It was a sad time. I lost about forty-five pounds in six months. The revelation, it has the effect of shaming you totally. It cuts you off from every other avenue of expression in connection with those you love. And there's a kind of doubleness, the first half of which is that you're ashamed about the defects of your personal, private behavior, and simultaneously you feel a profound, profound shame and divorce from the blessings of your relation with the person you love. A portion of that is the terrible sense of isolation and inauthenticity, knowing that if you ever get well, then you'll have to look at how utterly, and at some level viciously, you've wronged the person with whom you had promised to share your life. That final element of realization isolates you in your shame. It sequesters you so that you can never feel a genuine, unqualified love for the person you know you love. The more protracted and revelatory the confession is, the deeper, the more continuous the shame is, so as to make me inaccessible to anyone normal, including my own wife, and to compound my impulse to hang out in places of misdeed and treble my pain of various kinds in my relation with my parents and particularly my dad. You indwell with the feeling that you're a monster and capable of whatever's monstrous, and so there's nothing to impede your path to whatever kind of hellish behavior provides an externalized fantasy of what you think of yourself inwardly twenty-four hours a day. Toward the end of that last exposure, I couldn't take ten steps without expressing some form of disgust as a respite. That's when you start to worry about taking yourself out. It's a kind of jailing that feels permanent. It's a given. If you would pursue sobriety, that's the first thing you have to accept, and in another sense it's the last nail in the coffin, at least as you feel your situation when you're trying to get well. It's a bitter, bitter joke, the idea of getting well, when you feel so profoundly isolated and you feel that's properly so because of what you've done. I'm still on the Suboxone.

The show premiered in January 2012, and HBO picked it up for a second season after the first episode aired. In March, while we were shooting what would have been the second episode of the second season, a horse died. Two horses had died while we were shooting the first season. HBO paused production, and then HBO, Michael Mann, and I agreed to end the show. The official version was that it was canceled because those three horses died. They died in very ordinary ways—one got spooked by a rabbit and hit his head when he fell, one of their knees shattered, one broke its shoulder. We were working with the American Humane Association and following every protocol. PETA was doing a land-office business sensationalizing what happened and trivializing the love and care and effort of the people who cared for those animals and the spirits of the horses themselves. Whether or not you think Thorough-bred horses should be bred at all is a separate question, but they exist, and running is in their nature; it fulfills the deepest move-ments of their spirit. I think animals should be a part of art. To exclude them would be life-hating. Any living thing is subject to the laws of mortality.

I was relieved when the show ended, and Rita even more so. I suspect HBO was too—we were way over budget. Still, I found some dear friends while making it. Dustin is one. The writer Eric Roth is another. Eric's attempts at helping Michael and me work together were heroic. That's a blessing of the work we do, getting to know and love people we wouldn't oth-erwise. John Ortiz's character Turo Escalante was based on an-other horse trainer of mine, Julio Canani, and they got to know each other well. John got to California a month before the shoot so he could spend some time at the track, and he'd show up at Julio's barn at 5:30 in the morning. The first day Julio just ignored him. John was back the next morning. Julio said, "If you gonna be here every day, maybe you need a job." John was cleaning stalls, raking hay, filling the feed tubs. When Julio was first training horses, he was still selling carrots to other trainers from his trunk. He had to know John was tough, and he was.

Julio came to the track as a kid with his dad too. Julio's Pe-ruvian. His dad was imprisoned and Julio never lived with him, but every afternoon the chief of police would take his dad out of prison and they would go to the races together. Then he would drop him back at prison at night. His father had a full life. The fiction was he was under arrest, but in fact it allowed him not to have to hang with his family. He was a big, big co-caine dealer. So Julio never had a father except at the track. Then his mother finally took him and put him on a boat. She said, "If you stay here, you're going to be killed." I'm not entirely sure it wouldn't have been by his father. So there was an awful lot of unacknowledged rage and disempowerment and compensation for disempowerment. But along with that, there was joy. And Julio was just so, so good at what he did, and he loved his horses. I'd call him in the morning and ask about my horse, "Did she eat up? Did she stall last night? How was the abscess in her foot?" He just says the first thing that comes to mind. "Oh, she liking the new hay, and her goat." He and the truth have only the most flimsy and gossamer acquaintance. I hang up, and I know he's lied to me. He probably doesn't even know who he's talking to. But he allowed me the illusion that I was in control. There was such doubleness in him, and he was just the best liar I've ever met in my life. Some of the most fun I've ever had was when Julio was lying to me. John Ortiz got that too in Turo. When he'd say, "What a surprise," and he conveyed that it wasn't a surprise at all, that it was exactly the outcome he had planned, but there was joy in making the play, and anger that people still underestimated him when he showed how much smarter he was than they were every day of his life, that was it. If the show had gone on, there would have been some good stuff for John and Dustin to play together. But I'm glad Julio and John got to know each other.

I wish I had had more time with every one of those actors. Dustin and John and Nick Nolte and Dennis Farina and Richard Kind, Tom Payne and Kerry Condon, Jill Hennessey and Joan Allen and Michael Gambon and Ted Levine and Alan Rosenberg and Patrick Adams. Gary Stevens I knew pretty well from his days as a jockey, but I wish I got to spend time with him as Ronnie Jenkins. I especially wish I got to spend more time with Kevin Dunn and Jason Gedrick and Ritchie Coster and Ian Hart, who played the Degenerates, even though they pretty much got it all even without me there. What the four of them were able to play, what you were able to feel watching them was the truth the characters themselves didn't understand, that their real luck was the fact of their friendship. As individuals they have to lose—they win the big jackpot in the first episode, and over the course of the season each of them dissipates his quarter. But before they run completely out of money, out of some totemic impulse to memorialize the original victory, they buy the Cheap Horse, and thinking it's about the horse, they unite in friendship and their hearts open up. That process occurs in every one of the storylines in a different way.

Ultimately, in the overall construction of *Luck*, by pulling back from the individual storylines, as you feel the simultaneity of all these different spirits moving in a kind of concert, drawn and brought together under the same sky, you find there is a unifying principle in the midst of all the seeming disparity and pathology. Mr. Warren wrote of it when he was trying to describe Theodore Dreiser. Dreiser in his fallenness was appropriately born in Terre Haute, Indiana, on the banks of the Wabash. Mr. Warren described Dreiser and his brother as "particles beneath the great Mid-America loam sheet." But then the poem pulls back and asks, "Have you ever / Seen midnight moonlight on the Wabash, / While the diesel rigs boom by? / Have you ever thought how the moonlit continent / Would look from the tearless and unblinking distance of God's wide eye?" It looks as if the narrative is pathologizing everyone, but when you pull back and experience the story as a whole, you realize that what looks like pathological behavior is people vibrating according to their past experiences and the present coercions or liberations of their environment. The last purgation of fear is the impulse to see the story from any perspective other than that tearless, unblinking wide eye.

10.

Bleeding

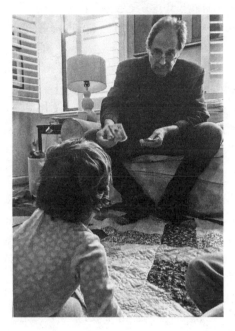

I NEEDED TO KEEP EARNING A PAYCHECK. We no longer had the same reserves to fall back on. But around when we began work on the second season of *Luck*, and subsequent to its cancellation, I noticed my mind started to slow down. It first began that I'd have difficulty remembering the full arc of a season without some help. Some of this could be chalked up to the fact that the kid was no longer a spring rose and I had a lot of city miles on me. I was lucky to always be surrounded by a group of intelligent, often younger, folks who could help me keep it all straight, but I know it was also somewhat worrisome for them. At that point, it was still easy enough to write off as a solid bout of aging, with maybe some depression sprinkled on top. But even as just a solid bout of aging, certain facts of mortality were being brought home.

I was fortunate in this period to take refuge in the work of William Faulkner. After *Luck*'s cancellation, that's where my attention turned. Having acquired the rights to some of his library, I began working on an adaptation of the novel *Light in August* together with my youngest daughter, Olivia. There is a passage where a character named Byron Bunch is riding his horse, mounting a hill, in the aftermath of having his heart broken and feeling rendered useless and unsure of the future he muses:

> Well, I can bear a hill . . . I can bear a hill, a man can . . . It seems like a man can just about bear anything. He can even bear what he never done. He can even bear the thinking how some things is just more than he can bear. He can even bear it that if he could just give down and cry, he wouldn't do it. He can even bear it to not look back, even when he knows that looking back or not looking back won't do him any good.
>
> [. . .]
>
> But then from beyond the hill crest there begins to rise that which he knows is there: the trees which are trees, the terrific and tedious distance which, being moved by blood, he must compass forever and ever between two inescapable horizons of the implacable earth. Steadily they rise, not portentous, not threatful. That's it. They are oblivious of him.

"Don't know and don't care," he thinks. "Like they were saying *All right. You say you suffer. All right.*"

It was a gift to have a repository for my efforts at that moment—as I have demonstrated, I am capable of directing them toward less than healthy ventures—and a special kind of blessing to channel them toward that work in particular, and shepherding the prodigious energy of my youngest child. Livy had in certain ways been shielded from me when she was a kid; she had such exuberance moving through the world and I think Rita wanted to make sure I didn't trample on it. That time, just after she had graduated from college, is essentially when we got to know each other, and getting that chance in its way revived me and kept me going in the years to come.

Television is unique among the arts in that it's pervasive and its demands are insatiable, and there are certain types of personalities that require what is demanding and insatiable as an organizing principle in their lives. There is so much static, so much noise that surrounds the process of trying to be heard, trying to be read, trying to have one's work seen, and it's crucially important that amid all of that noise and all of that static you align yourself with the simplicity of the essential act of writing. You have to show up, you have to give yourself to it, utterly, and you will find under those circumstances a blessing awaits you. The process is another blessing. The rigors of the process are such that the deepest impulses of our nature are revealed. The jungle will find out what you're doing there. That's kind of what television as a form is like too. It searches you out, and finds out what you're capable of, or what you're willing to settle for. Working in the medium requires an exotic combination of bravery and imagination—when you have a good imagination it can be very difficult to be brave.

I had been around for a while. When you feel yourself beginning the descent, you never know when something is going to be the last thing you do. You want to harbor your resources and try not to make a mistake. I became dependent on my collaborators in a new way in this period, and that dependence, along with a general depletion of energy, at times took shape as a kind of patience or willingness to make room for others that I had not been known for previously. I had started teaching when I was in my twenties, not much older than my students. When I was a younger writer I very much carried myself as the teacher, and I believe some of my colleagues found that grating or even insulting, and they'd be justified in that, at least some of the time. On *Luck*, they put me with collaborators my own age and it didn't go so well. After that, more and more often I surrounded myself with young writers who were the ages of my children. There was a mix of circumstances and motives in which I became somewhat more gracious, and they were willing to humor an old man and learn what they could from him.

I began working on a show with the producer Art Linson that we would eventually call *The Money* which used the trappings of a Murdoch-like family as a way to do *King Lear*. The media empire, the machinations. In *Lear* and in *The Money*, the tragedy is that this older patriarch doesn't want to let go. He doesn't know how to bequeath his power to the next generation and instead asks them to perform their loyalty to him in perpetuity. We were interested in exploring a family tragedy and a generational tragedy that has to do with the fate of a country (we'd all experienced too much of that already when we were working on the piece, and we've only experienced more, and to more disastrous results, since).

The mogul is James Castman, his company is VistaCorp. There were four kids. John the second-rate heir, the dutiful daughter Katherine who can't decide if she's in or out of the business, Greg the fuckup, and Teddy the mystery. Most of the characters weren't that likable, and what that imposes is an obligation that the play of the minds of the characters has to be compelling. But I was writing about an era of media and mass culture that I no longer was myself a part of. That may have been an issue. I know this all sounds like *Succession*, which came along a few years later. Don't worry about that. A number more than two writers have thought about the Murdochs and *Lear*. That's a great fucking show. My dear friend Brian Cox is remarkable in it, and all the kids are so alive and so wounded. They're making music.

In *The Money*, I barely ever left Castman. As I was working on it, I often found myself resisting settling into the family, resisting showing Castman settling into the dynamics of the family. I was working with two good young writers, Lucas Jansen and Amit Bhalla, who still work together. Amit was proposing that we have a dinner scene where we really lean into the family relationships, let them breathe for a minute. He said, "I wonder if it's better if there's this moment where they're all sitting around and they're just a family and it's devoid of the world outside. Maybe we do that thing with the home videos, where the four kids and Ruth watch and you see those dynamics and they can all laugh and be angry at one another at the same time. There's a respite from the plot."

I push back. "I have misgivings when I hear 'respite from the plot.' His life is an endless pursuit of plot, he flinches from respite from plot."

"But it's the thing that could be the saving of him—that's exactly his problem."

"His problem is the viewer's solution—the structure of the plot."

"Seeing his discomfort just sitting with his family, his necessity for plot has driven him away from his family and when he's there, as uncomfortable as it is, there's something warm and beautiful about it, and he can't appreciate it."

"His inability to participate—he retreats back into the plot. Lucius should be interrupting or he's on the phone with the Sheikh."

What became the main thrust of the series was Castman finding himself falling into an affair with the editor at the paper he buys in the pilot, and how that throws the family into disarray, and puts into question every structure and agreement they thought they were living by. But make no mistake, he's in love with his wife Ruth. He respects her and knows everything that she's given him. So what is it that unseats that? The surprise of it. The illusion of the re-capturability of youth, of spontaneity. In the story, I found myself reckoning with how a family goes on after the father fucks things up like that, and making the case to the younger writers I was working with that, even with the affair, Ruth would stay with him. She accepts whatever story he proffers accounting for his absence and indicates to the family that this is how it's going to be, that she's going to take him no matter what fictions are necessary. She tells her mother to shut the fuck up.

During this time, Rita was very much immersed in an effort to fix our financial lives, and week to week was still learning new ways I had been profligate, many I myself didn't remember. You'd have to be really crazy to sign away a portion of ownership in a network TV show to your Vicodin dealer. Don't put nothing past me. But having a lot of money and then losing it, especially in this country, it's better to owe millions than hundreds or thousands. There's room to maneuver. There are plenty of families, quite powerful ones, whose whole effort goes to that ongoing maneuvering. Borrowing against a mort-gage, against possible future earnings, and keep living as you are, with whatever self-loathing and misery is required to maintain the fiction. There may have been a world where we could have gone on like that a fair time longer, or in perpetuity. Maybe that was even the business managers' plan, once the ti-tles moved. But Rita, fairly, admirably, likes to feel the world around her is real, justified and accounted for, that it follows the rules in at least some ways, that it doesn't ask you to hate yourself. And so Rita spent years fixing the mess, turning her imagination to rebuilding our life in alignment with our cir-cumstances. She set up a payment plan with the IRS. We listed the house our children grew up in on Moreno, and the house on Martha's Vineyard. Rita sold her jewelry (which she never wore anyway, but I still bought). I was put on a forty-dollar-a-week cash allowance. She eventually got us to a new business manager. I can list these details not because I remember them but because they're in a court complaint that she would even-tually file, the basic premise of which was that I was so known to be untrustworthy that our business managers had had a legal obligation to Rita who was also their client to warn her and protect her against what I was doing. The case was settled out of court.

In the writers' room, talking about Ruth staying, I'd say, "Isn't that how we go forward? Isn't that how you show just how brave she is? My sense of Ruth is that she's so desperately hurt by Castman's behavior that to take any punitive action just makes her hurt too bad. She's outraged. She's unlucky enough to discover that under the right circumstances a person, includ-ing herself, is capable of tolerating anything."

HBO ordered a pilot and we shot it in the fall of 2013 in New York. Justin Chadwick directed. Frank Rich was a pro-

ducer, and he had a lot of insight into the world. Brendan Glee-
son played Castman. Nathan Lane played a newspaper reporter.
Ray Liotta was the rival mogul, Archer. Laila Robins was Ruth
and Rosemary Harris was her mother. John Carroll Lynch and
David Harewood playing Castman's lackeys, Harris and Cor-
bitt. Billy Magnussen, Morgan Spector, Ruth Negga, Mamie
Gummer, Andrea Riseborough, Tracee Chimo, Patrick Ken-
nedy, and Dominique McElligott. They all did great work. But
I was distracted—there were other forces at play that began to
weigh heavily on my mind, questioning my ability, my stamina,
and my health. While we were shooting I had a bout of anemia
and had to go in for blood transfusions. I had severe hemor-
rhoids and we believed the anemia was related to that. I was
losing a fair amount of blood each day. The general, accumu-
lating indignities of age are not for the faint of heart. Rita and
I would sneak off to doctors downtown but tried to keep it
mostly under wraps both because we didn't want to cause concern about my fitness to run a show and because I was embarrassed. This unpleasantness coincided with increasing instances
of confusion and memory loss, but we thought perhaps one
malady was spurring on the other. Unfortunately, they were
separate elephant fucks entirely. The great physician William
Osler said, "Nature is a very forgiving mistress, but she always
collects her due." Our eldest daughter got married in January
2014. I had to give a speech. I'm the guy who would rent a
theater when he didn't have a captive set of people to talk to,
but I did not feel good. I opened with, "Root for me." It was an
overwhelming moment, and one that stretched forward and
morphed as various realities came into focus. I had new needs,
and Rita in turn had new things to take care of, and that's how
we are together.

When the Brentwood house was first on the market, a

woman wrote to Rita and said she had driven past and then had parked and walked up and looked at the house and the yard and the trees and wanted to raise her kids there. That's what Rita had done, and it gave her pleasure to imagine this woman making a life there for her family. We sold her the house, and just after Elizabeth's wedding Rita and I moved to a smaller rental farther south. The family who bought the old house in Brentwood demolished it. The thing that upset Rita most wasn't the destruction of the house itself, or even that the woman lied, it was that she tore down the trees.

* * *

Not too long after that, HBO said they wouldn't be taking *The Money* to series. I turned to an idea about Boss Tweed and New York City in the late nineteenth century. He was a great thief and a great organizer. He helped build the city and ran the Democratic party within it, and then people came after him for being a thief. That show was going to be another mix of real people and some fictional ones, but you didn't need to embellish much. Victoria Woodhull and her sister Tennessee Claflin, their father turned them out as mediums, and they eventually made a mark of Cornelius Vanderbilt and built enough of a fortune to open their own firm on Wall Street in 1870. Vanderbilt, Roebling, Tilden, a lot of people who have beaches and bridges named after them were going to be in that show. Teddy Roosevelt's time as the police commissioner. It opened with Tweed in the jail where he would die, addressing a letter to his jailers:

TWEED

I am an old man, broken in health and cast down in
spirit. As to the charges standing against me, through

unpublished statements I've received some assurance
that the vindication of principle and purifying of the
public service are purposes you would have me serve.
Recognizing further resistance as a futility, offering
unqualified surrender and supplicating mercy, I
herewith submit my testimony—

I read that speech and a few more pages of the script we
called *Big City* during a talk with Matt Zoller Seitz for *New York*
magazine and people seemed to like it. That was the largest
audience that show ever had. HBO passed on it.

Writing was getting harder, but I found remembering a
day's plan or the day itself harder still. I was confused in ways
that even my formidable quirks could no longer explain. My
sleep was worse than usual. In January 2015 I went for a neuro-
psychological evaluation at UCLA and they confirmed what
Rita and I had suspected. I had dementia. Figuring out exactly
what kind of dementia you have is a test of one's tolerance for
uncertainty on top of the more rigorous one the disease itself
presents. It's hard to know. There also isn't yet a verifiably ef-
ficacious treatment for any particular type and so not too much
urgency to deducing further specificity. Plus I get claustrophobic and hate MRIs. My feeling sick all the time made Lewy
body dementia a viable candidate. When I would eventually
get the full scans a few years later, they could see the plaque
built up in my brain and gave me the diagnosis of "Probable
Alzheimer's." The final confirmation only comes at autopsy.
That doesn't make too much difference. Once you're in the
general dementia ballpark, you're playing a very long game.
There's no winning, there's just hanging on.

My agent John Burnham was resolute. He knew I wanted to
keep writing and so he figured out how I could keep writing. I

began work on an adaptation of Peter Matthiessen's novel *Shadow Country*, which tells the story of a sugar planter in Florida named Edgar Watson who was eventually killed by a group of his neighbors. The whole work is about trying to figure out who this guy was. It tells the story from his neighbors' point of view, then his son tries to reconstruct it years later, then Watson telling the story himself. There was a time when Jeff Bridges was going to play Watson and Scott Cooper was going to direct and I was writing it. It would have been a limited series, which I hoped might assuage any concerns HBO might harbor about my sticking to deadlines and my own about my ability to remember the plot. We wrote five episodes. HBO decided not to move forward with that one either.

You feel it when the collection of work that has never been made accrues weight. The fact that *Big City* and *Shadow Country* were not made, and *The Money* was not picked up, was not lost on my psyche. The weather gets a little cold when your last few things haven't sailed. You start looking over your shoulder, second-guessing yourself, questioning your value and worth even more than usual. This doubt was compounded by my diagnosis, which seems only fair.

But then, not too long after they passed on *Shadow Country*, in the summer of 2015, HBO started talking about doing *Deadwood* again, as a movie. I had told Richard Plepler, who was then CEO, and my producer Carolyn Strauss about my condition. I don't know if anyone else at the network knew or not. In January of 2016, they gave me the go-ahead to write it. Len Amato was the head of films then and he's the one who ultimately said yes and made it happen.

About a month later, *The Hollywood Reporter* came out with an article about my gambling problem and how I'd put my family into debt, only five or so years after the fact. My family had already pretty well come to terms with it by then and so in a way things coming out in the open had a certain relief, or at least release. Rita in particular had feared she would be criticized, either for allowing me to get so out of hand or for filing suit or for staying with me, but that never came.

At that talk with Matt Zoller Seitz, he had asked if people should abandon all hope of *Deadwood*'s return, and I said yes. I truly believed it wouldn't happen. There are cynical or ironic ways one can interpret any sequence of events if one wants to, and that is all the more tempting when major corporations are involved. But when I was given that chance again, to go back to *Deadwood*, I primarily experienced it as an extraordinary gift. It felt to me to be an enormous kindness from people I had known and worked with for decades, and in this instance the fact that they were network executives also motivated by commerce or some possible turn in public perception was all the better. When one feels oneself losing ground it is nice to feel that people with skin in the game still want to back your play.

11.

Mornings

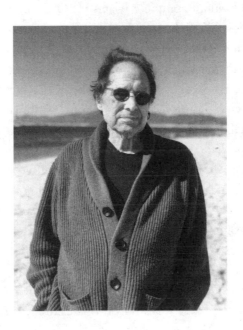

I HAVE NEVER BEEN RIGOROUS in exercising the part of my brain that dealt with the logistics or material facts of day-to-day life, but the muscle that lets me explore the logic of a scene or story and walk around inside it is one I have exercised daily, near on fifty years. The chance to organize behavior around a different reality is art's great blessing, and this was especially true in my state and circumstance. Working in earnest on the *Deadwood* movie script offered the chance to go to a world with a manifest organizing principle and structure that was familiar to me. The world's rules, how to question the soundness of a scene or a character's behavior, the interior logic of things—despite how diminished I felt or how slowly I feared I was moving—I chose to believe I could still make sense of it and move the material forward. There was a part of me that feared I wouldn't be able to, or that I would complete it and HBO would say no again. Nothing I could do about that. All I could do was work.

We started by looking at some of the old notes and manuscripts generated when we thought there would be a fourth season. Pretty quickly it became apparent that that wasn't where we were going to find the truths of the story we were going to tell at this juncture. It was a different time. Over ten years had passed. Where could we begin?

I began to imagine Al had another brother who came to camp and it fucked Al up. I was imagining that Alma had also returned and that Martha, Seth, and Alma were once again navigating their triangle. There was a stakeholder named Wallins who was murdered by Hearst's men, and Seth tried to avenge him. Soon enough I realized Wallins had to be someone we already knew and cared about, had to be Charlie Utter. But all of 2016 I was working on this draft with Al's brother. Early in 2017 Carolyn Strauss gave me a very good, very clear note to get rid of him. I came back and asked some of my other collaborators how much it would screw us up to implement that and, quite upbeat, they replied, "Oh, not at all, in fact we've already taken him out." I was the last to realize. The elephant in the room is Swearengen's mortality. How is he dealing with the recognition of his mortality and what is he going to do about it?

I wasn't good about getting back to Buffalo. Made it once every couple of years maybe. I had a tendency to get depressed when I was there, so we were judicious about it. Sometimes I would have a trip planned and then I would start having chest pains the night before my flight. Bob and my mom accepted it. But in 2017, as I was working on the *Deadwood* movie, I went back twice. My mom was ninety-seven. She'd had dementia herself for just over a decade. Bob had managed her care throughout her illness, found her a home that could meet her needs as they increased.

The first time I went back was in April. Elizabeth was pregnant and had a sense that my mom wouldn't live to see her child, but she wanted to tell her about it, and so we went together. I had to have a travel handler escort me from when Rita dropped me at LAX to where Elizabeth could pick me up in New York so I wouldn't get lost. My mom already had eight great-grandchildren by then, with whom she was very close, but this would be the first from my line. When we told her, my mom turned to me, asked, "Are we happy about this?" She wasn't sure how old Elizabeth was, maybe she was still seventeen. Elizabeth jumped in. "Yes, I'm thirty-three. I'm married." My mom smiled. "In the right order. That's wonderful then." She proceeded to tell us which of her fellow residents she thought wasn't very bright.

In June, my brother called to say it was time to come say goodbye. Mom was in hospice, the hospice my brother had run and where she had volunteered. Rita and I went, and we were there for the weekend, but Mom held on. She died once I got on the plane home.

* * *

Driving had become an increasingly iffy proposition for me. With some regularity, I lost the keys, or the car. Rita found and rented a new office around the corner from our house that I could walk to, a little bungalow house with a kitchen and bathroom that she outfitted with my dictation setup and a bed so I could nap. The connections between Al's condition and my own were not lost on anyone. There were some days I would look at the pages and ask who wrote them, only to be told that I had. I was incredibly lucky and grateful to have a team of collaborators around me who made the telling of this story and the doing of my work possible. Regina Corrado came back to help, to keep all the threads in mind so I could focus on the stitch. I leaned on her, and others. In that sense, it was the greatest distillation of the process of writing in which I have ever engaged. In encountering the materials, one felt that nexus of experience hospitable to more storytelling, that there was more to know, more that would be discovered if one was willing to risk the possibility of an ineffectual repetition. Finally one felt that those themes as organizing facts could be made friends. This was the conversation with my assistants Allie DiMona and Brittany Dushame one day in September 2017, over a year and a half into work on the script, as I worked through a revision:

"I think that—I may be absolutely mistaken in this—but I think we need to defer to Al as the organizing force in the resolution of this story because Al is the most pragmatic and unprincipled of all of the positive characters. Look up 'the good is what works.' Swearengen is the archetype of that perspective. And the proper organizing dynamic of the storytelling ought to be located in his person. He has the most energy as an organizing force and yet his physicality is diminishing. And that's a tragic, invisible irony. And you have to play scenes in which he says to Bullock, the spirit of what he says is: 'My son, we are going to hold hands walking into this situation. I hurry to assure you that this will not be a permanent condition. But for the moment we need to be as brothers. You have to be my instrument. You have to break the law, because I am weakened physically. And it's only if we augment each other that we are going to be able to accomplish our purpose.'

"Now if we can accept as a principle of storytelling that the viewer is to be gratified by Swearengen enlisting Bullock as his right-hand man, that is a pleasing combination to the viewer's sensibilities. Because you get the pleasure of watching Swearengen be unprincipled and Bullock disinfecting Swearengen's unprincipled impulses. Now what are some of the situations that have to be addressed by that combination? Bullock and Swearengen acting in concert. What is Swearengen's problem in this episode?"

"He's dying," Allie says.

"He's weakening. And what is his greatest source of pride? His strength. His shameful secret is, he's losing his strength. As a pure pragmatist, the pragmatists believe the good is what works. It doesn't matter if it's morally right or wrong. If it works, that defines it as good. That's Swearengen. Now he is confronting the tragic paradox that every human being confronts as time goes on, which is the diminution of power and its corollary perception that 'might makes right.' What he is having to look at is the fact that he can't get things done on his own. He needs to work through Bullock. He needs to work through the whores. He's got Trixie to deal with. All these things are diminutions of his ordinary power. The story that we're telling is the story of individuals coming to deal with the fact that, of themselves, they are incapable. That they have to collaborate with others in order to get their goals accomplished. At one level, this is a story told from three different perspectives about the accepting of limitation. About the fact that Swearengen doesn't have the muscle that he needs to be a muscle guy. And that Swearengen has operated through force up to this point and now his force is diminishing. And how is he going to have to collaborate with others? Who is he going to have to use? Can he accept the fact, as any man must as time goes on, that he can't go for the gusto anymore? Essentially, this is a series of vignettes dramatizing the overarching truth, which is 'of myself, I am nothing.' Now let's look at the different stories from that particular point of view. What illustrates the power of the principle of cooperation? Which of our stories can fit into that, can be viewed from that perspective?"

* * *

HBO started talking to the actors, seeing if they could get schedules worked out to shoot the next fall. That was an enormous undertaking, because the actors were almost all busy, and they had to move through whatever feelings they had about the series's end, and its potential return, and their lives and careers since, to decide whether they could walk through the thoroughfare again. The person who had the most reservations about coming back, and he said so himself, was Tim Olyphant. He wasn't sure he wanted to put that badge on again. In March 2018, he told an interviewer he didn't think the movie would happen. We had some good, long talks that spring, and Tim had a lot of thoughts about where Bullock should be at this moment, in his relationship with Al, with Martha. Every one of them made the movie better. He came to our house in May—just me, him, and Rita sitting in the back house with the dogs.

Tim says, "It's this tricky thing, trying to balance—he's always been the guy who's sort of carrying the weight. He's a heroic figure, he's doing the right thing, he's got the best interest of the town in mind, but it gets problematic in the movie if everyone else is having way more fun. I think we need to look for opportunities where you feel like he's having fun. I say that knowing that he's still gonna be driven and he's still gonna be acting for the good of the town but he's going—"

"That's absolutely right."

"Otherwise, why bring him back? I think you wanna bring him back to realize he's got the world by the balls, and now he's up against it and he's got all these things that're happening, and his best friend just died. He's going to kick ass and take some names. If he has to go outside of the boundaries that he's used to, that's fine, he's gonna go outside some boundaries. This is the way we're gonna play the game now. We're gonna play by their rules. That becomes fun. I think that's where we want him to live."

"That's it."

"I wanna go and really lean into it, to be able to say, 'I'm gonna work my tail off so when it comes on the day it's gonna be effortless.' I don't know if I should say it out loud, there's a part of me that really wants to come and be like, 'Okay, the revelation of the movie was Bullock, was Tim's performance. It just went to a whole other level.'"

During the first run Tim often joked that he didn't know how he ended up the straight man. Like Bullock, he hadn't closed in any articulate way with the predicate of his gift. I think he halfway thought he was getting over, that he was getting away with something. And so when he told me out loud what he wanted, that he wanted people to see something different in Bullock and in him, I was proud, and I was ready to serve him, to act as a vessel to deliver that wish. He wasn't standing back. He was grabbing at something to take the weight. The pleasure for him was the discovery of his sincerity, of wanting to choose something with his whole heart. That ultimately became Bullock's pleasure too, his and Martha's and Al's discov-

ery that he had sincerely chosen this town and this life, and he
was enjoying himself. And people did see it.

When he left one of our talks that spring he said, "I'm
around, I'm available. I will get as involved as much as you'll let
me or allow me, but I don't want to be intruding where I'm not
helping. Lean on me, call me. I'm here."

That's when I knew we were going to make it.

* * *

That fall, we were back at Melody Ranch, in the mud again.
Dan Minahan, who had directed four great episodes during the
original run of the show, came on to direct. Gregg Fienberg was
producing again. Most of the actors, we had stayed in touch.
Paula, Robin and Earl and Kim and Keone, Michael Harney,
they came to see me fairly regularly. Lunches with Ian. Most
everyone had a fair sense of what my condition was like going
in. We all knew it wouldn't be the same. We had a table read,
and the first lines in the script belong to Jane. "Ten years gone,
'proaching that selfsame hill I thought to lay me down and rise
no more." As Robin was about to say them, she sort of gasped.
Then she says them, and her voice breaks, and in the saying she
brings back this whole world, in an instant. If you go back to a
place that you've lived, you feel an instinctive flinch. You think,
"Jesus Christ, I won't know a single soul here." And then it
turns out you still know everybody. That's a very gratifying, rewarding experience. One risks describing it as redemptive.

I couldn't do what I used to do, rewriting on set, improvising, talking philosophy. We didn't have the time or budget, but
also I just couldn't. What I did instead, with help from Rita and
Olivia and Regina and others, was prepare a speech to read at
the start of each shoot day to set the stage for the scene and
prepare our spirits however I could.

On day four, for a scene with Dan and Johnny, W. Earl Brown and Sean Bridgers:

"Dority and Burns were and are our chorus. Each is a transitive presence, effectuating the passion and thrust of the material. It's taboo in both of their feelings to talk about Al going to die, and once they expose the subject, they feel guilty, sinful. Living under Al's rule isn't always easy and admitting that he's sick and admitting that he's going to die is admitting Dority and Burns are going to have to figure out life without Al. The idea that the most potent figure in life, the father, might pass, is anathema, and yet they know on some level it's an inevitability. They're scared shitless about a world without Al. Who would they be in that world, how could they be in that world? Part of that fear is rooted in the reality that they half might like it. There's freedom in that, and that's terrifying. By broaching the subject, hitherto taboo, they begin to deprive Al's passing of some of its power. To give it voice is at some level to disempower it. Giving it voice is another way of saying, 'I'm afraid,' and another way of saying, 'I love you.'"

On day eight, for a scene with Trixie and Jewel and Al, the last thing I said was, "The truth is you don't have much say on whether people love you for you. That's the miracle. It just happens."

We were always talking about love making that show, about the strange ways it shows itself, every single day. The pure joy of meeting up again with old friends and jamming. We played together so beautifully. To borrow a line I gave Alma, it was "a dream come alive to draw breath." There were days I could only make it on set a few hours, a few I didn't make it to set at all, but every single one made me so grateful. I knew I could trust my collaborators. I could give it to them now. Every person was heroic. Molly Parker was making a show in Canada and she would fly down on weekends to shoot her scenes and she was so tired, she would sleep in her dress on the ground. My old friend Franklyn Ajaye came from Australia so that Samuel Fields could once again show how dangerous and heroic it can be to simply exist. Geri had had surgery not long before and she was in pain, but she came back to be our Jewel. Ian would give me a kiss every day. Earl would play guitar and sing.

* * *

Bodies, after a period of exertion, knowing they've completed a task, have a tendency to break down. "Oh, we did it? Great, because I'm spent." College kids always get sick after finals. Something like that happened after we finished shooting, while Dan was still in the edit. My confusion got worse, what had been a loose grip on reality became more untethered. Mornings weren't so bad, but with dementia and Alzheimer's the late afternoon and early evenings are notoriously worse. They call it sundowning. In early 2019, for the first time, there were moments when I wasn't sure who the people around me were. There was a night in January I turned to Rita and asked, "Is Rita dead?"

"No, I'm Rita. I'm right here."

"I should call Rita. Where's my car?"

"We share a car now. I can drive you if you need to go somewhere."

"Would you dial a number for me?"

"Who do you want to call?"

"Judgy. Do you have Judgy's phone number?"

"He's dead."

"Aw, he's not dead, I just spoke to him a few days ago. You've got to go with me on this."

I'd ask her what to wear to the event we were going to when there was no event. I'd make her drive me to the bank, say there was six-hundred-fifty thousand dollars waiting. I'd tell her I wanted to separate and ask how much money she needed to sever our connection, would five hundred thousand do the trick? She took notes on her phone so she could report back to my doctors and to Bob.

But mornings were still better. With help, I could still work in the mornings. It was around this time that I wrote what would become the first pages of this book, dictating in the room in the back house Rita had made into an office. The one a block away had become too far, we'd let it go.

The movie aired at the end of May. Everyone had worked so hard to get us to the finish line, and we got there. During the press run, in large part to account for my absence from it, we announced my diagnosis publicly. The implications that had for my future work prospects weighed on me, but there would have been no way to pretend my condition wasn't real and getting worse. I couldn't have pulled it off. We trusted Matt Zoller Seitz to break the story, to tell the world on our behalf. He had visited the set and spent time with us. So did his frequent collaborator Alan Sepinwall, who first made his name writing *NYPD Blue* recaps when he was a college student. The day he came my granddaughter was there too. Mark Singer, who had written a profile of me for *The New Yorker* back during our second season, wrote another piece where we talked about how I was doing and feeling at some length. I described some of what was happening to me: "It's a series of takings away. And there's a subsidiary category of shame, at not being able to do things . . . More than anything else, one would like to think of oneself as being capable as a human being. The sad truth, imposed with increasing rigor, is you aren't. You aren't normal anymore. You're not capable of thinking in the fashion you would hope to as an artist and as a person. Things as pedestrian as not being able to remember the day. Sometimes where you've been. There have been a couple of times when I haven't been able to remember where I live. And then there are compensatory adjustments that you make in anticipation of those rigors, so that you can conceal the fact of what you can't do. It's a constriction that becomes increasingly vicious. And then you go on."

The evenings took darker turns that summer. I'd ask Rita to drive me somewhere but not say where we were going. "We may be killed doing this. Do you have a gun?" I'd ask her to take me to the police, but she was worried that if we went, I'd say something that would get me committed to the psych ward. I'd say things to her that asked a lot of her patience and grace, even knowing the circumstances I was in.

"Can I not go through it tonight?"

"Through what?"

"Telling the truth about stuff. I've never hurt anyone. I've never done anything like that. I've never killed anybody. I've never done anything that most people would consider evil. Don't think me a bad person because I've done bad things."

"What do you want to confess?"

"Sins of the heart."

I started forgetting that I wasn't supposed to drive anymore. I'd try to steal the keys. I'd yell at her for them. One night, I was walking out of the house, insisted I was leaving, and I fell face-first on our front brick steps. A lot of blood, very confused.

I was hospitalized, and the doctor told Rita I needed to be in full-time care, that the way we were living was no longer safe for either of us. In October 2019, I moved into the memory care unit at an assisted living facility not too far from our house. Rita set up my room, got me a bed and furniture and put her paintings all over the walls, set up the cable. There was a cat named Mignonne that would visit me. I'd stay there at night, and she'd come get me during the day so I could still work in the back house. I had begun collaborating on a limited series about Johnny Carson with Lauren Stremmel and Brittany Dushame and kept trying to work on this book. I couldn't hold the whole structure of something in my head, but in the mornings I could talk about character, I could work on scenes or lines, try to identify the dynamics at play in a given moment. I wanted to stay productive.

In November, Rita went to New York for the birth of our second grandchild, Olivia's son Morris, named for my grandfather who tried to go over Niagara Falls. Sometimes those weeks she was away, I'd think she had left me. I'd call and she'd explain the circumstances again, that she loved me and all was well. In February 2020, Rita took me out for the weekend so we could go to our son Ben's wedding in Santa Barbara. All my children and their friends and my grandchildren were there, and my son was happy.

Then it was March 2020. The virus came. I didn't get to see my family or anyone else for a long time. It wasn't good. Didn't know how to use the phone. No one to dictate to. Would lose the legal pads Rita sent me, mix up the manuscripts she'd drop at the front desk. I missed everybody so much. A lot of asking if it was four P.M. so I could get my Suboxone. There was a brief window, which Rita tells me was October, when we got to see each other. I met Ben's son Hank then, when he was three months old. Then the window closed. I got sick. Mostly I was confused. I thought I was wanted for murder. There was a plastic seal in my room. People coming in in bubble suits. Sometimes I thought Rita was angry with me, that we were divorcing, that that was why we were apart. I'd talk to my family and say, "I pray we get to be together again." Some days I'd ask Rita to marry me, tell her I wanted us to have children. I'd sit in my room and look at Rita's paintings on the walls, try to get lost in them. She'd drop off snacks. She'd drive by and wave from the window three stories below. Have someone come in to tell me she was there and waving. Lose a year and don't know what you lost. The cat moved into my room. Mignonne stays with me full-time now. Rita says she adopted me.

Things opened up, and my brother got sick. First they thought it was his heart and they gave him a stent, but he didn't feel any better. In April they realized it was liver cancer, and it had gone to his lungs. We would talk on the phone. A few of those video calls when I was with Rita, but I didn't like those. I didn't want to be another thing for him to put on a face for. When he was sick, he would explain to his kids what was happening to his body, to make sure they understood. He said he'd do a few tests, to help everyone come to terms. He worked with his own hospice to set up his pain management. He died in June 2021. I didn't get to see him. None of us knew how to manage getting me there, both of us sick in our different ways. Elizabeth went to the funeral. I had written a few words for my brother that she was going to read. I called her fifteen minutes before the service with line edits. She was sitting there with my nieces and nephew and Bob's widow, Linda, and taking the edits. They renamed the hospice in Buffalo for him. He was as good and kind and sweet a soul as I believe God ever made. I miss him so much.

There's a passage of Ernest Hemingway's *In Our Time* that describes a pair of soldiers wounded and likely dying together in an alleyway among the greater chaos and destruction and bloodletting in the aftermath of a battle. One, his face turned toward the sun, addresses his partner: "Senta Rinaldi. Senta. You and me we've made a separate peace." He qualifies, "Not patriots." He notes the comings and goings and stretcher-bearers up the street. Hemingway wrote, "Things were getting forward in the town. It was going well." A separate peace made. A facet of human nature is our ceaseless will to go on, even in the face of unspeakable pain. Its going on is life's organizing nature.

* * *

Two voices. One and two. Me and Rita.

"So we're talking about an expansion of the premise involving sports journalists, in particular horse-racing journalists. If the sports journalist was old, seventy-six, like I am, and he carries a book, and if he tries to sell himself to the younger reporter as a man of repute and more than a little bit, but not a tremendous amount, of reputation and power, and the kid initiates the examination of that premise—that may put too much of a burden in the viewer's mind on the old man's role because the old man is kind of hanging on by his fingers. If the old man were to have a friendly relation with the reporter, who would be not old but thirty-seven, say. He can see the finish line." That's me.

"The old man's a bookie?" That's Rita.

"The younger man would be like thirty-seven years old and what generates his seeing the finish line is a flagellation. His fears about his incapacity prompt him to really unwarranted fantasies. The old man is going to ensnare him. He's dismissing the life of a gambler as viable, but he keeps coming back to it. The kid wasn't born yesterday, he has this certain sophistication, and he understands the old man's running scared. And the journalist has endured failures of nerve himself in contemplating how to proceed. There's a mix there I'll know how to choreograph. The old man is looking at the finish, but he still has a certain reputation as a journalist."

"I thought the old man was a bookie and the thirty-seven-year-old was a journalist."

"Both."

"Oh."

"I think that the relationship between the old man and the kid hangs around the margins of larceny and disreputable cons. You don't want to make it too neat. I'll have to work on how you choreograph the seduction. The old man can see that the younger fella is attracted to the idea of being a gambler as an identity rather than an occupation. Under the guise of simply befriending the younger gambler, he orchestrates—it's a web of wounded psychologies juxtaposing and in their woundedness drawn to each other. It's a disastrous juxtaposition but most juxtapositions are disastrous. How do you react?"

"I think it's good. It sort of reminds me of *The Main Chance* with Eddie and Abe Chait."

"That's right. That's right. I didn't think of it until this moment."

"And it also sort of makes me think it's your younger self and your older self."

"Good for you."

"But I think it's good and keep going."

"There's a female reporter and journalist who is the instrument of the advancement of the story, who sees versions of herself in both of the other characters. She's going to try and become sexually involved with the younger reporter in order to seduce, and that triangle plays and it gets more destructive as it goes on."

"Maybe she's using him to do a story on the bookie."

"Oh, that's good. I think that the old man is on an accelerating path of self-destruction. He's retired from being a bookie only to recognize how vacuous and empty that life is as a parasite and so he is made to confront—the old man is made to confront—the sounded void of his life. And he tries to resurrect the possibility of becoming respectable in his own idea of himself and other hangers-on at the track. You get a kind of a circus effect. Once you generate a dynamic you can usually extend and populate it. The old man discovers the willingness to do something as emotionally and psychologically destructive as, you know the expression 'turning out'?"

"Mm-hmm."

"He's looking to turn out the younger of the three and set them against each other and orchestrating false jeopardies and that's a manageable choreography."

"Is the old man trying to scare the guy out of the life that he led?"

"I think that he's trying. He never had the nerve to pursue as destructively and as baldly what this kid is doing. But as the story progresses the old man, in sight of what another writer called 'the sounded void of his life,' he tries to compensate, tries to save the kid."

"What makes him understand that, the sounded void of his life?"

"He doesn't. What seems to shadow a good deal of the storytelling is a general sense in the characters of an encroaching malignant reality, that they're vulnerable. They would never admit it, but they don't feel quite equal to the combat. And they've got all kinds of tics to protect themselves, or to accommodate their fear. It's gonna be work but I think it's doable work. I would invite you to work on the writing. It'll be a hard ten weeks but that's not the end of the world."

"Okay."

"We were working on this, and my brother died a couple of weeks ago."

"I know."

"Did I tell you that?"

"I know, I'm so sad."

"Very brave."

"I miss him a lot. I mean, I talked to him a lot."

"Did you?"

"Yeah. I mean, he would help me take care of you, your care, so we talked a lot."

"He was a good soul."

"Mm-hmm."

"Pray on it and make sure, because it'll be demanding."

"I know. I will."

"But there's no reason that you can't get a credit as a writer. Go home. I'll give you a ride. Did I drive you over here?"

* * *

It's awful being crippled like this. Hobbled. It's a hobbling. It's an accumulation of the ineffectual. I can't remember what I meant to do. Honesty dictates that I evaluate it to its detriment in comparison to what I used to be able to do. There's a cumulative solitude which is onerous. It just weighs on you, and it doesn't take much on a given day to tip over. *Who am I kidding?* There's a momentum toward giving up as a way of saying, "At least don't let me embarrass myself." I work as I'm able, as long as I'm able, but the mandates of futility point in a different direction. What is in prospect is an abject loss of control, of human prerogative. I hate to lose my dignity. I miss Rita more than I can say, and the children. Sometimes I feel that I'm walking among strangers.

I imagine different configurations of characters at the track, or in an office building. They're usually old. They're strangers to the deepest drives of their natures. The question that one asks oneself is whether they're so alienated from their own inner lives that their lives are living them. Their fear is that they can't develop a predicate understanding of themselves and so they find themselves driven without any comprehensive understanding of what's moving them. They have glimpses of it but they're of an age, as I am, that they feel their inner lives are an inaccessible mystery. They find themselves driven by forces they can't locate in a way that mobilizes understanding and behavior. The fear that they live by and into is that it'll stay, that the forces that drive them will control their actions without their being able to identify and comprehend these drives. They've reached an understanding that it's increasingly unlikely that they ever will, which is an invitation to despair. The challenge that the work needs to encounter and confront is the growing fear that it's beyond, that whatever these wounds may be, that they're too potent to find a constructive way to engage them. I share with them the growing suspicion that the struggle is futile, that they're too late, but still trying to locate and focus an understanding of how he can proceed so that he can live his life. If he can find out what the controlling elements of his life are—but the likelihood is that he's not going to make it. How do you bring yourself to encounter that or those truths and still behave constructively? And the growing realization of the struggle's futility and that his life is living him and what that means. The truth comes home that this life is real and it's earnest and it's for all the marbles. You can do more than you think you can. The least desirable of all the possibilities is to die stupid, to die without having recognized what was at stake and what the possibilities might have been in the situation. You minimize a character if you don't see him aware of those stakes. This is my life. I'd hate to die a fool. This is why shows about the elderly get such huge ratings.

I think about Johnny Carson, about the Carson show, imagine scenes with him thinking out loud, but in fact he's talking to God. Jack Benny as God. In the dynamic of the storytelling, he yields more and more—he gives himself to the premise of who he's talking to. "You know, not for nothing, there have been times when you were a little slow on the uptake." The process of communication is emotionally exhausting to him, he's waning, and the idea of God becomes more and more accessible. And he postulates God as his old friend. Johnny tries to work him, tries different kinds of jokes on him. He has the impulse to try and bribe him, and then he says, "I'm kidding. That's nuts! What do you need money for?" As the relationship develops, "You're not how I pictured. Of course, no one made me the authority. You are who you are. Between you and me, how bad was it when Christ died? Oh, He was the Word made flesh. That's the problem! Always been mine!" There's something tentative in the impulse to grill God about what's really going on, and if it's Benny, he can say back, "This is just how it works, I don't know. Ask someone else!"

If the narrator were asked to announce a kind of overview, if he were to ask himself, "Why am I doing what I'm doing? *What am I doing?*" the sense of order is provisional and there's a degree of desperation. "Why am I doing this? Am I talking to God?" Who is he talking to? That's what he's asking himself. "I got a right to ask the question, everybody's got the right. The big thing that concerns me is, am I an asshole?" That's what's fueling this process, his being impelled to self-examination. Who do you think he is thinking of?

He might pull back from a just-completed paragraph, "Who

am I talking to? I must think that there's somebody listening."
What do you think of him? Do you respect him? What entitles
him to your respect? Is that going to get him out of town?
That's what he's asking himself. Someone's at the door. Some
people have bad souls. Who the fuck am I talking to? Why am
I doing this? Is it gonna get me out of town alive? Is He listening? Apparently I feel like I'm talking to somebody.

The question of the listener's identity is fundamental. Who's
listening? Who are these people? Why am I concerned with
what they think? Why do I have a right?

I choose to believe. The worthiness of getting up and reaching out, the act itself undertaken against doubt. Maybe I'm
wrong. Shoot me. So many different manifestations of the
choice to act as if. I make no claim to certainty on any ground.
I make my only claim to worthiness on the ground of will and
choice. I will act as if my being is worthy and thereby purchase
its worth. It's shifty ground. He's got a microphone and he's
doing a show. You know Johnny Carson can slide into this.
That character is haunted by exactly the same questions.

Let me say from my heart: Don't give up on mass culture.
Contribute to it. Break your heart in trying to make it better.
Our species is in a fight for its life and nobody says the decision
is going to go one way or another. Put your bodies and your
spirits up. I used to have this dream of setting up a school with
all my shows that never got made, call it either the Writer's
College or Big Wave Dave University. Anybody who wanted to
work on them could come, and I'd work with them, and the
classes would be filmed and put on the internet. My sole stipu-
lation would have been that the writers also become teachers.

All you can ask for out of life is to get into an environment
where you try to do your best. The mistake, which is one that
I make a lot, is not to spend enough time appreciating how

lucky you are. It goes so fast and it's so easy to have an inauthentic relation to it, which is: *I'm so tired. Jesus Christ, I just
finished one and here comes another.* Life will let you do that. It's
important to communicate the joy and pride that you feel.

One manifestation of that is paternal connection. I can't tell
you how many hundreds of times I walked into one or another
of the kids' rooms and just wondered at the absolute miracu-
lousness of what transpired. Their mother, my wife Rita, who
did all the heavy lifting, brought to the process of child-rearing
an imagination and a specificity and determination and candor
and gentleness that was just something beautiful to behold. I
remember when I was a kid, when I was first starting to drink
and do other stupidities, always assuming that the natural condition was to experience a barrier between oneself and the others one came in contact with, and that that was a given. The
miracle was to watch Rita be absolutely present and move
freely between her imagination and the kids' imaginations—
like there was a larger creature that had been created in which
the four were completely integrated parts. It's a curious thing
to say, but to watch it felt like you were stealing. It was so beautiful, the sweetness of it. In particular her generosity, and the
gift freely given, over and over, was just extraordinary to see.

Now we are getting to experience some of those joys again
as grandparents. Our eldest grandchild, Lou, has adopted
toward me a sort of casually pleasant tone. She calls me Dave
and thinks I'm funny. It's just happening. The younger two
grandchildren are boys, Mo and Hank. With each of them, you
become absolutely present. That's a lot of upside for me at this
point. I don't have to think about everything I don't remember,
don't have to pretend I know what they're talking about. We
just play. Everything is an adventure and a delight and a surprise, an opening up, and that's a big gratification. We all get to

participate. We are all on the ride. When I look at my grand-children or I hold them, I can feel that it's only my individual strength that is subsiding. The strength in the family, in the species, and in the whole beating heart of the universe hasn't subsided at all.

To the extent that we have progenitors or become them, when we're blessed with children, nature builds into us the im-mediate sense of a special imperative connection, but it does not simultaneously ask the question, "Are you ready? Are you healthy? Because it would be better for the child if you were healthy." Nature doesn't allow that. It's life on life's terms and nature's own time. My relationship with my dad was an enor-mously complicated one, and with my children in turn, but that's another way of saying I and they were born with DNA. The particulars of the complication, to insist upon their uniqueness would be to misunderstand the blessedness of being able to experience it.

I still hear voices. I still tell stories. There are those in my head and another in my throat and others in my work. There is the voice in my wife's head and the ones in my children's heads. The deepest gift I think an individual can experience is to ac-cept himself as part of a larger living thing, and that's what we are as a family. Shut the fuck up, Dave. I still hear that voice too.

I hurry to acknowledge an incertitude about what I'm say-ing. I tend to be hospitable to not having a certain sense of how things are going to turn out, to be willing to entertain the pos-sibility that they're not going to turn out at all. That incerti-tude is a proper part of the process, to know that I don't know the answers. Sometimes I don't even know the right questions, only that there's a particular kind of urgency in connection with a series of events. That urgency doesn't tell the truth about the events, it only tells me, "Enter here" and "Go here next." That can be an invitation to self-indulgence. I have to be willing to risk that, to entertain that as an organizing truth. The process of storytelling, when it's wrung from the heart, is a process of discovery, and self-discovery, and that has remained true with this work at this time.

It seems to me that a life lived all the way up embraces the dangers of failure, and is undertaken nonetheless. When I sit down to write, that's an outcome I have to be willing to embrace. It's a privilege and a blessing and a pleasure to come with whatever limitations are imposed to encounter the possibilities of telling a story. The older you get, to the extent that foolishness doesn't shape your behavior, you know that you've been given a gift and you try to honor it.

I don't know the answers to the questions that have brought me here. But I'm willing to walk with that incertitude and not be afraid, or to be afraid and walk with my fear. I'm always walking with a particular kind of darkness when I'm in the process of composition, or drawing breath. I try to think of it as ultimately producing a friendship. A friendship with the darkness, and a belief that my incertitude is itself the seed of friendship. There's a familiarity that develops out of that acceptance. I'm facing challenges and discontinuities that are new, but they aren't complete strangers—the uncertainty, the fear, they have been companions before. What am I talking about? It's all the same thing. I'm making the decision to believe that this process of storytelling, begun again, will have a formed and happy result. That may or may not turn out to be an illusion, but one at least has the solace of knowing one entered with a willing heart.

Acknowledgments

To the many, many people I have worked with, worked for, took drugs or pursued sobriety with, gave or owe money to, or shared a meal with, I love you all and I'm grateful that our paths crossed. You are the people I met on the river.

I will always owe an enormous debt to my late friend Steven Bochco for taking a chance on me and seeing what we could do together.

Jeff Lewis has been my friend for over fifty years now and brought me to the work that would change my life.

Mark, Fran, and James Lytle, thank you for our time together and letting me share Judgy.

Bill Clark has walked with me down the road and made my life so much richer. Thank you for sharing it with me.

Billy Finkelstein was the first reader for this and much of my writing. It's a gift to have a friend who makes you laugh and tells the truth.

Judd Apatow and Eric Roth, Michael Harney and Paula Malcolmson, our lunches have been a source of joy. Thank you.

Richard Plepler and Carolyn Strauss, thank you for your friendship and support. I will always be proud of the work we produced.

To Linda, and to Linda and Bob's children and grandchildren, thank you for sharing him with us, for carrying on his kindness and understanding, and for making him so happy.

Regina Corrado has been a constant and welcome presence throughout this project, interviewing people at the outset, always kind and supportive and knowing. I also want to thank Brittany Dushame, Micah Sampson, Jesse Allis, and Lauren Stremmel for their help in putting this together.

Thank you to all my former assistants for your patience and your effort. I am so grateful to each of you for making my life possible.

The Beinecke Library at Yale holds all my papers and those of my teachers too. It's a place that's helped me in the process of discovery and rediscovery many times over.

Ben Greenberg at Random House helped shape this from the beginning, constructive and encouraging the whole way through. Thanks to Jenn Joel, a supportive presence throughout this project. Their faith that this could be made it so.

It is a rare privilege to be able to work with your children and I've been blessed to have had that experience with all three of mine. On this project, my deepest gratitude goes to both my daughters. Olivia got the ball rolling, believing we could do this when the rest of us were less than certain. Elizabeth helped me give it its final form and made sure the work knew itself. They organized material from many years of writing tapes, lectures, and script notes which helped enormously as my memory flagged. These days it's hard to make new memories that stick but what does stick is the feeling of being loved and this endeavor has allowed me to finally and gratefully accept that feeling.

Each of my children has built their own life and family. There is no greater final gift than knowing your children move free from obligation to you, that whatever you get of them is of their own volition. Elizabeth, Ben, and Olivia—thank you, I love you, and I couldn't be prouder of you. Lou, Mo, Henry, and any grandchildren yet to come, same goes for you.

And finally, thanks to my wife, Rita, who has shown me love, commitment, and patience in practice every day for forty-five years.

About the Author

* * *

DAVID MILCH graduated summa cum laude from Yale University, where he won the Tinker Prize. He earned an MFA from the Iowa Writers' Workshop at the University of Iowa. He worked as a writing teacher and lecturer in English literature at Yale. During his teaching career, he assisted Robert Penn Warren and Cleanth Brooks in the writing of several college textbooks on literature. His poetry and fiction have been published in *The Atlantic* and *The Southern Review*. In 1982, Milch wrote his first television script for *Hill Street Blues*. Among other credits, Milch created and wrote the shows *NYPD Blue*, *John from Cincinnati*, *Luck*, and *Deadwood*.

About the Type

* * *

The text of this book was set in Janson, a typeface designed about 1690 by Nicholas Kis (1650–1702), a Hungarian living in Amsterdam, and for many years mistakenly attributed to the Dutch printer Anton Janson. In 1919, the matrices became the property of the Stempel Foundry in Frankfurt. It is an old-style book face of excellent clarity and sharpness. Janson serifs are concave and splayed; the contrast between thick and thin strokes is marked.